Ethel's Story

Bioenergy Book One

Michael Yanuck MD PhD

This book is dedicated to

Ethel and her family

and for Cathy and the children

To the Reader

The names of most of the people in this book have been changed and certain information that might identify them disguised.

Bioenergy is a technique that can be learned, and it is my hope that this book will serve as your first step towards acquiring this skill.

Michael Yanuck MD PhD

INTRODUCTION

Ethel worked in the Office of Student Affairs where I went to medical school. She was quite simply the most beautiful person I had ever seen.

Tall and graceful; when she walked she flowed; and her smile radiated a delight in people and tangible feeling of care.

I was shy and hollow chested, with big inquiring eyes, rounded shoulders, and unsure expression.

I tried to remedy my shyness by teaching CPR.

Ethel arranged the classes.

When I'd appear at her desk frustrated and disheveled, she'd look at me as though to say -

"Hi, Mike... How are you?... What's the matter?... Are you okay?..."

My classmates referred to Ethel as 'the most beautiful woman in the world' -

I thought I was just another admirer.

Still, whenever I ventured into the Office, my eyes were drawn to her.

Waiting to see my guidance counselor -

She'd be sitting at her desk -

Eyes directed downward -

Faint smile on her lips -

Looking as though captivated -

Wondering what she was thinking -

"Mike, what brings you here?!"

Leaping from the chair, I'd go racing into my counselor's office -

Struggling to remember what I'd come there for...

An elective was being offered in reading EKGs -

I stood in line at the Office, waiting to sign up -

My classmates talked amongst themselves as I carelessly looked about the room -

Ethel was rising from her chair -

A memo in her hand -

She walked to the Registrar -

Smooth, effortless strides that flowed one into the other.

I looked on, admiring, feeling privy to a wonder.

Then, as she passed in front of the Dean's Office, her image began to fade -

It was as though her form were changing -

Dissipating -

Becoming one with everything around her.

All else remained unchanged -

The Dean's secretary sat intently staring at the papers on her desk -

The ambient sound of talking was the same.

Smiling, I stepped back, leaned against the counter, and subtly shook my head -

I would never understand, I thought...

At the end of my third year of medical school I was awarded a prestigious scholarship, and worked to develop a vaccine for cancer at the National Institutes of Health.

The work went well at first.

Then, six months into my research, I suffered a leg injury.

Doctors gave me little hope, and said I could expect chronic pain for life.

I sought other forms of healing, and, ultimately, found a clinic where I was not only treated, but trained in their techniques.

At the end of six years I completed a dissertation detailing my research.

But what I'd learned went well beyond its pages...

Leaving Washington DC, I drove back to medical school.

Crossing the bridge to Streeport, a vision of Ethel - smiling and floating - came into my head.

The thought of seeing her filled me with exhilaration, and I wondered how it was I hadn't thought of her in all these years...

Arriving on the Midland campus I proudly marched to the Office.

But opening the door I had to step out again because everything inside was changed.

"Can I help you?" said the woman at the front desk.

"Yes, I'm looking for Ethel James."

"She isn't here anymore. There were some personnel changes a few years ago, and she left."

"Oh."

I turned my head away, and hid my hurt expression.

"Is there something I can do?"

"No, that's okay."

The woman stared at me, then sent darting glances to her colleagues.

I moved to the door as though in slow motion.

Outside in the hallway still-life portraits surrounded me.

"Things have really changed," I thought.

I walked out into the midday heat and humidity -

I didn't think I'd see her again...

Michael Yanuck MD PhD

Part One

CHAPTER ONE

I called my former instructor, Dr. William Brand, and asked if I could spend a few weeks on his service?

"Yeah, sure, Mike. We meet at noon at the Medicine Team A office on the sixth floor. Why don't you show up then..."

Cool and unpretentious, his voice lingered as I put down the receiver...

Six years ago I had been floundering on the wards.

Medical training was not at all what I'd expected.

Where I'd envisioned a center motivated by care and compassion, I found, instead, a boot camp, where patients were dispensed with like a bothersome commodity.

My instructors (called 'attendings') struck me as oddly detached and unavailable -

Rather than inspired, they left me consumed in the question of what their motivation was.

Dr. Samuel Irving was my first attending.

Large and rotund, his body fit him like a clanky barrel, and his lazy eye drifted, so you could never be sure which he was looking at you with.

On my first day he was discussing a patient with stomach problems -

"I don't know what we're gonna do for this guy," he said. "Nothing seems to help."

"Dr. Irving," I perked up, "I read an article about using erythromycin to stimulate the intestines. Could that help this patient?"

He turned to the two interns.

"What do you guys think?"

"I wasn't familiar with it," said one.

The other shrugged his shoulders.

He asked the chief resident.

"How about you?"

"Never heard of it."

Dr. Irving turned on me.

"Rule number one! - Never upstage your residents and chief!..."

The following day I was asked to present on rounds -

"The patient is a forty-six year old..."

I looked up from my notes -

Dr. Irving was grinning to the residents, making quivering gestures with his hands.

"In conclusion..."

I dropped my head, and stared blankly.

Dr. Irving responded with a single emphatic nod.

"That was good!" he said.

"The next time, though, I want you to look at me!..."

Dr. Irving was scheduled to give a lecture.

I'd been on-call the night before, and in the warm, darkened auditorium began to nod off.

Halfway through I resolved to stay awake, and got up from my chair, walked to the back and stood for the remainder of his talk.

That afternoon we made rounds -

Dr. Irving stood in front of a patient's door, and gave a short discourse on tuberculosis.

Afterwards, he gave me a hard look.

"A lot to know," I said.

"Well, maybe if you hadn't been sleeping during my lecture you'd know this stuff!"

His expression was severe - As though I needed to be severely reprimanded.

A moment later, though, he appeared strangely embarrassed...

The next day my chief resident pulled me aside -

"Mike, yesterday was Dr. Irving's last day on the service. Dr. Brand will be taking his place. We're all gonna meet with him at noon."

He grinned.

"He's a good-OLE Texas boy. You're going to like him."

I had the image a man in cowboy boots - Sneering, and eyeing me like a pathetic sissy.

"Oh, no," I said.

"Mike, Dr. Brand isn't that way," he insisted. *"He's a gentleman..."*

At noon we sat in the small confines of the Team G Office waiting for Dr. Brand.

I was in the back, hunkered over my chair.

"Don't worry, Mike," one intern said.

"It isn't going to be bad," said the other.

The door became ajar, and a man's face peeked in -

"Are you guys from Team G?... I just wanted to make sure I was in the right place. I'm Dr. Brand..."

His voice was subdued and soft-spoken, and he moved with slow, careful, noiseless steps -

He picked up a heavy chair from a corner of the room - lifting it with ease - and then sat with the rest of us -

"You guys want to go through your patients?"

He was tall and gaunt, but his manner was so gentle he struck me as almost small -

"What do you think of that?"

His tone and bearing was like no attending I'd ever seen -

There wasn't the hint of anything intimidating or overbearing about him -

He treated us as equals - Genuinely interested in what we had to say.

I looked at him.

He wore Rockport shoes - The same as I did.

Our eyes met -

His expression was mild and unassuming, and radiated a gentle glow.

I, on the other hand, was bubbling over - Fighting to suppress my smile, and outward expressions of relief, exuberance and joy -

I had found the mentor I'd been searching for...

CHAPTER TWO

I strode to the entrance of the Claude Ray General Hospital wearing my short white medical student's jacket for the first time in six years.

I had just passed through the doors when a security guard called me back.

"Excuse me, sir. We'll need to see some identification."

"Oh, sorry," I said. "It's been a long time since I've been back here. I guess things have changed a little."

I took out my wallet, and showed him my six-year old medical student badge.

"That's a good one!" he said with an amused smile. "Go on through..."

As I made my way through the corridors a feeling of exhilaration swept through me -

Everything felt exactly as I'd left it -

The stairs I had rushed up and down on - The laboratory where I'd carried samples - Rooms where I'd taken care of patients - Some who died suddenly - Others who perked up and recovered despite my thoughts that they wouldn't survive.

I'd forgotten how much I'd delighted in being here -

Now it was all coming back to me...

On the sixth floor I waited in the Team A office.

One by one the members of the Dr. Brand's team trickled in.

"Hi, I'm Mike. I was a student with Dr. Brand six years ago. I'm just back from doing a PhD..."

The team was assembled, and we were all waiting for Dr. Brand.

Then the door swung open -

4

The first thing I saw was a pair of pointed cowboy boots.

Dr. Brand?!

I got up to greet him -

"Hi, Dr. Brand. Nice to..."

"Whoa!" he called out. "You've got white hair!"

He took a step back, and nearly doubled-over in a fit of nervous laughter.

"I thought I was the only one who'd aged in this place!..."

CHAPTER THREE

I got home late that evening.

I'd been assigned a patient, and the work-up kept me at the hospital till dark -

My clinical skills came back easily -

As though I'd never been away...

It was a still and humid night -

I put on a bathing suit and went down to the pool.

Resting by the water's edge I thought about the day's events -

Being with Dr. Brand was as riveting as ever -

His way of speaking - simple and direct, intense and incisive - reverberated inside of me.

Still, I couldn't help the feeling that something about him had changed -

During afternoon conference he sat in the very front of the room with the other attendings, and kept his back to the rest of us.

Six years ago he'd sit in the middle, and engage the residents in friendly banter.

Now the feelings he exuded were ones of impatience, hostility, and disdain.

I sat in the back - Wondering why the change?

Then, a look of horror gripped his features -

It was as though he were staring into something frightening and overwhelming -

With nowhere to run, and no one to turn to -

Having to face this terror alone...

Laying my head back in the water I breathed a sigh of relief -

Finishing medical school wasn't going to be difficult at all, I thought. I would cruise through my remaining rotations - No problem.

Still another part of me felt sad and alone -

If I didn't believe in this stuff anymore, why was I here?

The years following my injury I had come to lose faith in conventional medicine -

I was on different path now -

One centered on healing, and not just treating disease.

But who would employ me? I thought. What credentials did I have?

There were reasons for coming back - Completing my medical training was a stipulation of my PhD.

But how would I cope with doling out treatment I no longer believed in?

Perhaps I could say, "I'm not the one writing the orders - I'm simply the student - Here to learn and observe."

But the emptiness lingered -

If my heart is in it, why am I here?

I got out of the pool, and prepared for the next day...

CHAPTER FOUR

The next morning we met again in the Team A office.

I presented my patient.

Dr. Brand looked over, and gave a nod of his head.

"Are there any other patients to go over?"

"No, that's it," the upper level said.

"Alright. Let's go have a look at them."

Dr. Brand got up, and the rest of us followed him into the corridor.

I felt light and happy -

I was another day closer to completing my degree -

This was going to be a breeze.

Caught up in my thoughts, it wasn't until we'd gone down a flight of stairs that I noticed Dr. Brand seemed to be leading us away from our patients.

What are we going down here for? I thought. All of our patients are upstairs.

On the fifth floor he led us to a room on the Pediatrics unit.

I stood holding the door for the others, and was the last to go in.

Dr. Brand was in the far corner of the room, talking with a female patient.

She lifted her gown, and he proceeded to press his stethoscope to her abdomen.

She looked at him intently - Her eyes thoughtful and child-like.

She appeared small and delicate, and the way her hand rested on her gown reminded me of an expecting mother.

In the dimly-lit room I felt a certain admiration -

There was Dr. Brand - Tall and handsome - My ideal in a physician -

And this woman, who seemed to sense that, and willingly availed herself to his care.

Then, maintaining the diaphragm of the stethoscope against her abdomen, he removed the earpieces and looked at me.

"Taken a listen to this, Mike."

I shot back a look of surprise.

"The patient has an abdominal bruit," he said. "The others have heard it already because I brought them here once before. I just wanted you to have a chance to listen."

A scintillating feeling took hold as I eagerly made my way forward.

Standing opposite him I took the earpieces.

"Whoosh... whoosh," the sound of the bruit.

"You hear that, Mike?"

"Yes, I do."

Then, an ethereal voice rose up, and seemed to echo from all four corners of the rooms -

"I know Mike."

I looked up, and met the patient's eyes for the first time.

Her nose was flattened, and I wondered if someone'd hit her - And if it hurt?

But the kind, delighted smile never wavered, and the caring, inquisitive soft brown eyes drew me close.

Who was she?

Faces of patients sprang into mind -

None matched this woman.

Where did I know her from?

I prided myself on my memory -

Even if it were six years I should be able to remember.

I peered deeper, unwilling to give up.

Then, her features became liquid, and congealed and coalesced in my mind's eye -

"Oh my God!" I said. "This was the most beautiful woman in the world!"

Behind me the members of the team laughed approvingly.

Ethel dipped her head, closed her lips around her pearl-white teeth, and subtly shook her head.

"Where did the two of you know each other from?" Dr. Brand said.

"Ethel worked in the Office of Student Affairs."

"You worked at Midland?!"

"I worked there for twenty years."

"You didn't tell me that," he said with nervous laughter. "How did you wind up at a place like this?!"

"I left a few years ago to start my own business. That didn't go well, and, since, I've been working in a dermatologist's office... Their insurance couldn't cover me because of my previous diagnosis of MS [multiple sclerosis], so I've had to go through the county hospitals and clinics."

"Gosh." He looked up dumbfounded.

"So nice to see you, Mike!"

I wanted to embrace her.

"I'll be back later, Ethel," I said.

"Okay."

Dr. Brand looked perplexed, as he held the door for the rest of us, and we filed out into the hall.

"I would have never guessed she worked at Midland," he said. "She's been coming in and out of clinic for weeks... She's had a lot of pretty non-specific symptoms - Loss of appetite - Nausea and vomiting - Comes and goes, off and on - Haven't been able to get a handle on it yet.

"She'd been seen in clinic, but between the different teams and attendings, they really hadn't been able to tell her much - You know how that goes.

"Anyway, when I saw her in clinic the other day and heard the bruit, I got her admitted so it could be worked-up..."

I was hardly listening.

"I've found her," I thought. "I've found Ethel. I've found her!"

"There's got to be more going on there," he said. "It's strange..."

CHAPTER FIVE

Long flowing curtains encircled Ethel's bed when I went back that evening.

Drawing them back she was sitting, covered warmly in white blankets - Her expression like a small child in an unfamiliar place - Unsure and fascinated at the same time.

"Hi, Mike."

"Hi, Ethel. I brought you some food... It's rice and steamed vegetables. I thought it would be more gentle on your stomach than the food they give you in the hospital..."

"Oh, Mike, you didn't have to do that..."

"I wanted to, Ethel. I thought it would be good for you."

"As it is I've already eaten. But your food does look delicious."

"It's easy on the stomach - That's the main thing," I said. "For a long time I had stomach problems, too, Ethel. In just a couple of months I lost twenty pounds."

"Oh, you did, Mike?"

I thought she didn't believe me - like a grown-up listening to a child's tall-tales.

I stopped talking, and looked away.

She went on looking at me, though, waiting.

I stared out the window at the sunset -

"When I was growing up, I used to spend my summers in New York.

"My mom would pack us up - my brother and me - and send us out there.

"We'd go to summer camp, and in the evenings ride bikes to the local high school.

11

"There was always ice cream in the freezer - We'd come home and make malteds..."

The light in the room was dwindling -

"I love being back in Streeport. I love the nighttime. It's so quiet and peaceful - Not like the east coast, where it's cold, and always feels like there's something biting at you..."

Ethel's face was smiling - Eyes glowing in the dark - Pearl white teeth shining - Looking at me as though enraptured.

"Ethel, I brought this plate and utensils - May I leave them with you? I think they're a lot nicer than the ones the hospital gives you - It might make the food more appetizing."

"Are you sure you don't want this back, Mike?" she said. "It's a very pretty plate."

"No, Ethel. I want you to have it..."

The next day on rounds Dr. Brand talked about research -

"There's a lot we don't know, though," he said, "and things can be missed. I remember my wife one time - right after she'd delivered our son - kept on complaining of a problem with her shoulder. I didn't know what it could be, so I didn't say anything. Finally she says, 'Why don't you examine me?' Sure enough she had winging of the scapula... That's right, paralysis of the long thoracic nerve. What caused it and why it should be related to the pregnancy - I have no idea...

"Mike, you had something like that... Did they ever find out what it was?"

"Yes... Myofascial pain and dysfunction."

He depressed the corners of his lips.

"Never heard of it. How long did you have it?"

"Pretty well the entire time I was away from Streeport."

"You see!" he laughed. "You come back to Streeport, and you're cured!..."

CHAPTER SIX

"Oh, I have to take you guys out to lunch," Dr. Brand announced casually on the last day of service. "Where do you feel like eating?..."

We went to an Indian restaurant in downtown Streeport.

"So, Dr. Brand," said one of the medical students, "how did you arrive at the Claude Ray?"

"Oh, that's a long story. I was working in research for a while. I came out of Midwestern with a lot of honors, and wound up with a pretty sizeable grant from the NIH.

"I worked at the Sabin Institute. When I went there, I thought I was going to spend the rest of my life behind the research bench... I was doing the kind of work Mike did... Working with oncogenes.

"But it was really tense - I didn't like the competitive feeling in the lab, and there were people doing what I considered a lot of questionable science...

"I gave it up... Yeah, quit... I even sent the remainder of the grant money back to the government.

"I went back to Streeport - No job, didn't know what I was going to do. One of my old buddies asks me, 'So, you think you're too good to work here?' I told him, 'Nothing doing', and got a job at the Claude Ray the next day."

"Where were you from, Dr. Brand?" I said.

"Here... I was from Streeport... I grew up in the shipping lanes with my mother. We were poor, poor."

"What about your father?"

"I didn't know my father."

Then, he smiled, and looked at me with a sly expression.

"You didn't want to know my father. He was a gambler and a lady's man. Take my word - You didn't want to know him."

"Did you have a step-father?"

"Yeah. My mom remarried this guy. We didn't get along much. One night I got home late - I was boxing at the time and working out a lot at the gym - He comes into my room drunk - Says 'So you think you're pretty tough - Let's see how tough you are'.

"So, I knocked him down, and never went home again."

"Do you still box?"

"I used to. I stopped just recently."

"Why did you stop?"

"I got hurt... I was boxing this young guy. He wasn't very good. I guess I hurt him pretty bad.

"Anyway, after I'm through fighting this guy, his trainer comes up to me -

"'Okay,' he says. 'Now I want to fight you.'

"So I'm fighting this guy, and by this time I'm really tired - All I can think of is 'When am I going to get out of here?'

"Finally, the bell sounds, and I drop my hands. I'm thinking 'Whew, glad that's over.'

"Then, he nails me with a punch right in the center of my chest... Yeah, broke a couple of ribs.

"A few days later I develop this accelerated cardiac rhythm - I never knew when it was going to go off... Yeah, I'd be sitting down at morning report, and, then, right out of the blue, my heart starts racing."

"Does it still bother you?"

"No. I've got it under control now."

I hesitated.

"When you were growing up, who did you spend your time with?"

"I spent most of my time with a couple of Spanish families in the neighborhood."

I looked away -

"For myself," I said, "I had something of a self-imposed poverty placed upon me.

"My father grew up poor - He made his own way through college, and insisted I do the same...

"And, where love was concerned, I always seemed to have to find that outside my family - Usually in the homes of people much less fortunate than ourselves..."

"Yeah! I think that's right!" he laughed. "I mean - They've got a lot of love."

I directed my gaze downward, unreconciled.

"Last week one of the Spanish families I told you about made a surprise birthday party for me," he continued.

"Did you go to their home?"

"No, they came over to our place... My wife arranged it... Oh, she's a doctor... She has a practice in northwest Streeport..."

CHAPTER SEVEN

Ethel's chart was lying on the table in the nursing station when I went back that afternoon -

I sat, and flipped through its pages.

An ultrasound had been performed earlier in the day -

The analyses were a page long -

This blood vessel clotted - That vessel clotted - Extensive damage to the spleen -

I read and re-read it, shaking my head.

Dr. Brand came gliding into the ward -

"Did you hear about Ms. James?!" he said. *"I had no idea it was going to be this tragic!"*

Before I could speak he was clear past me...

"The way I see it, Ethel," I'd told her the night before, *"pain is trying to tell you.*

"Too often in conventional medicine, we suppress symptoms, instead of addressing the underlying cause - We give patients a pill, rather than tell them, 'You're going to have to make some real life-altering decisions if you're going to get past this.'"

Ethel had looked away -

I collected my things, and got ready to leave her.

Then, she fixed her gaze on me - Eyes shining - The very core of her beautiful being radiating out at me -

"I wish you well, Ethel," I said. "On your journey into health..."

"It's just a few vessels," I told myself. "She'll be okay."

I stood alone in the hallway.

"What have I been saying?..."

CHAPTER EIGHT

Friday night I was on-call with the Neurology service.

Ethel had left the hospital a few weeks earlier, and I hadn't spoken to her since.

As I made my way to the intensive care unit, I casually read the names of patients posted on the doorways.

"... Tanya Sykes ... Vanessa Roberts ... *Ethel James?!...*"

I stepped back, and peered through the glass.

Ethel was standing next to a bed, folding her belongings, and putting them in a small valise -

Her movements had a strange furiousness about them - Like she were shaking about, trying to disperse a swarm of biting flies.

"Hi, Ethel," I said, stepping into the room. "How are you doing?"

"Oh, fine, Mike. I'm about to leave... Yeah, I had another bout of nausea and vomiting... Oh, I'm pretty much okay now, except that I have this pain right here in my back. Mmm-mmm. I don't think I ever had back pain like this before."

Her voice was anxious, and she continued to fidget.

"I have to go to the nurse's station to call my daughter, Shon. She'll be picking me up soon..."

Another medical student walked in behind me.

"Hello, Ms. James," she said. "I just wanted to say goodbye."

Ethel hugged her.

"Oh, thank you, Dora. Thank you for all the help you've been..."

I accompanied her to the nurse's station.

The gown hung limply from her emaciated figure -

She looked like she only existed in two dimensions, and, turning sideways, would disappear.

17

At the counter she leaned steeply and supported herself as she talked into the phone.

The back pain is really bothering her, I thought.

Overhead, I was being paged -

"Medical student, Mike Yanuck, to the emergency room. Medical student..."

I backed out of the ward - My eyes fixed on her...

CHAPTER NINE

The next day I met Dora in a hallway behind the emergency room.

"Hi," she said. "Were you following Ms. James?...

"The surgeons want her to come back to the hospital. They saw a spot on the CT of her pancreas. Originally they thought it was hallow and represented a pseudocyst. Now they think the mass might be solid.

"They also went back and reviewed the CT of her abdomen. Her liver had been previously read as normal, but now they think they see a couple of suspicious areas there that could be masses..."

Pancreatic cancer.

Of course.

The abdominal bruit and blood clots -

The nausea and vomiting and back pain -

It all fit together.

"I hope not," I said.

My insides were shaking -

"It's one of the few cancers where the spreading cells actually infiltrate the nerve sheaths and directly irritate the nerves. It causes severe back pain - The worst known to medicine - Worse than kidney stones..."

Dora stood frozen.

"Thank you, Dora. Thank you for telling me this."

She didn't respond - But followed me with her eyes as I left the hallway...

I wandered through the hospital.

On the fifth floor I saw Dr. Brand on rounds with his new team -

He was talking to a patient in the hallway, then turned and marched past me without a word...

A fellow student on the Neurology service saw me.

"What's the matter, Mike?" he said

I told him.

"Maybe they're wrong!" he insisted. "Surgeons say that about a lot of patients, and they usually all turn out to have pseudocysts.

"I saw it all the time when I was working on Surgery at the VA. The cysts can be drained, and the patient does just fine..."

CHAPTER TEN

A Sunday morning two weeks later saw me striding out of the Claude Ray -

I had just completed my rotation in Neurology, thereby fulfilling the core requirements for my medical degree.

Walking along side me was my upper level resident John Wang.

John had majored in philosophy, and said I was someone he could talk to 'because of my advanced degrees.'

Despite having spent the past two nights on-call, he was still bristling with strength and energy.

There had been difficult times between us - I didn't like how he referred to patients -

But, now, our tour of duty behind us, we walked into the mid-morning sun laughing and smiling - Our heads held high.

Just then a small voice called out -

"Hi Mike!"

I looked over.

Ethel sat on a cigarette-stained cement bench wearing a hospital gown.

John followed me over.

"They did a biopsy of my liver," she said, "and found out that I have cancer.

"So, it's a relief to finally know what I have."

'Relief'?! I thought. "You have cancer! Don't you know how terrible that is?!

"I hope now that they can do something to cure it - Now that we know what I have..."

Her voice maintained its polished tone, but her speech began to ramble.

"Ethel," I said, "John here has been up the past two nights, and I want him to get some sleep."

I looked at John.

He just shrugged his shoulders.

"I'm alright," he said.

"I'm going to walk him to his car," I said. "I'll be right back."

"Okay, Mike," she said, smiling.

John cupped her hand in both of his.

"I wish you the very best."

His tone and bearing were so dignified I felt small in comparison...

At the parking structure we shook hands.

"I just wanted to tell you who much I appreciated all the training you've given me," I said, "and how impressed I was with the long hours you put in on the wards."

"Well, you do what you have to do," he responded gruffly. "All these scum-bag patients you come in contact with while you're doing your training, you have to figure, 'They don't matter'. What matters is you're at the top of the ladder. By the time you get to the level of training we're at, you're on the superior rung of society..."

I went back to Ethel.

"So, did you say goodbye to your resident, Mike?"

"Yes, Ethel."

"He seemed like a very nice person."

I hesitated.

"Yes. He taught me a lot."

She searched my eyes, smiling.

"That's good, Mike!"

I nodded.

"Hey, Ethel," I perked up. "Did I ever tell you about the time we went horseback riding, and my mom stepped on horse poop?"

A beguiling smile stretched across her features.

"No, Mike, I don't think you've told me that one yet..."

CHAPTER ELEVEN

"...So I'm sitting there at the kitchen table eating my spaghetti, and all of a sudden, out of nowhere, my mom says, 'Michael, stop that!'

"'Stop what, mom?'

"'Stop going, *'Mmm.'* Every time you bite into your spaghetti you make an *'mmm'* sound.'"

"Because you really liked it," Ethel interjected, smiling.

"Oh, yeah! My mom made the best spaghetti and meatballs. It's about the only thing I ever remember eating - I guess because I liked it so much.

"Anyway, I say, 'Oh, sorry, mom.'

"So I go back to eating my spaghetti, and I'm being really careful not to go, *'Mmm.'*

"But the next thing I know, she's saying, 'Michael, you're still doing it!'

"'Doing what, mom?'

"'You're still going, *'Mmm!'*

"So she tells me to get up and go to my room."

"But she let you take your dinner, right?" Ethel asked with gleeful expression.

"Oh, yeah, she let me take it with me..."

Just then, Dr. Bryce Hood entered the room followed by the members of the Oncology service.

The mood of the team was somber.

"This is Dr. Bryce Hood," the fellow announced. "I told you yesterday he would be by to see you."

"I know Bryce."

Dr. Hood stood, head bent, at the foot of the bed.

"Hello Ethel."

A former Midland student himself, my first impression of Dr. Hood had come six years ago when he stood in front of my class, and, without notes, delivered a lecture that covered such a wide range of topics it left us in awe.

"He's a walking encyclopedia," whispered the student next to me.

But there was something else - The way he peered up nervously at the class - that left me feeling that behind his prolific memory he had something to hide...

"There are a number of treatments that we can try, Ethel," he said.

In his monotone voice he recited a list of options.

Ethel listened intently -

"I'll consider the things you've just told me," she said in her *poised and polished tone. "And get back to you when I decide..."*

"Finally, before we go," he said, "I want to examine you."

The others took a step back, except for a single female student who would act as chaperone.

He glanced in my direction -

"Draw the curtain."

I sat looking on -

"Draw the curtain."

He repeated himself without irritation -

"Draw the curtain."

I gazed over at Ethel -

"Draw the curtain."

Her eyes were closed, directed downwards, and smiling -

"Oh."

I jumped up and jerked closed the curtain...

A tall, gangly student walked over.

"Did you know her?" he said in a solemn tone. "I knew her, too.

"Hi, I'm Brian. I'm in the combined MD/PhD program. I'm just coming back into the wards. I entered Midland a couple years before Ethel left..."

"I knew her too," he said...

Dr. Hood left the room and wrote a note in Ethel's chart.

"Dr. Hood," I said, "can I ask you a few questions?"

"Yes, except that I'm on my way back to The Marymount Hospital."

"I'd be glad to walk with you..."

We left the Claude Ray, and crossed the street to The Marymount.

"I want to get her on an experimental protocol using an anti-tumor drug called nitro-camptothecin," he said. "A group at St. Jude's has reported achieving remissions with it in some of their pancreatic cancer patients..."

"So what have you been doing?" he asked.

"I just got back from completing my PhD," I responded. "I did my work in cancer vaccine development."

"Did anything become of it?"

"The animal studies became the basis for a FDA-approved clinical trial. As a matter of fact, the first patient who entered the study had metastatic pancreatic cancer. When it got on the cover of Time we became swamped with pancreatic cancer patients - None of them did very well..."

At The Marymount we parted at the elevator.

"If she has any problems," he said, *"bring her to me...."*

Ethel was waiting when I returned -

"Mike, people with my illness - They do get better, right?"

I hesitated.

"I suppose it's possible, Ethel."

"But they do have treatments for my kind of cancer, though?"

"Yes," I nodded, my eyes averted, "they have treatments for it."

She looked at me with a blank expression...

At the bus stop I sat on the curb and took out a pen and paper - Bus after bus passed me by -

The short white jacketed figure returned...

CHAPTER TWELVE

The home I lived in was like a dungeon -

Into it had come a sinister figure who'd managed to take hold of and dominate my wife.

He'd drilled a burr-hole into her skull, and sealed it with a metallic knob; then, while I was away, insert an agent into her brain that made her have convulsions.

"Your wife had another one of her fits," he said. "She wasn't able to finish her chores, so she has to work longer."

"You can't do that!" I said. "I'll go to the police!"

"Now you wouldn't do that, would you?" he responded with sly smile.

I walked across the groove to a neighbor's -

All the time feeling the cross hairs of a rifle fixed on my back.

I was met by two affluent friends -

"Surely it isn't as serious as all that?" one said. "Is it really necessary?"

Before I could reply, I awoke -

My heart pounding out of my chest -

I have to affirm who I am! I thought...

I went to Ethel's room at the hospital -

But the bed was stripped, the dressers empty, and she was gone...

CHAPTER THIRTEEN

Ethel's chart was in a collection bin -
I took down her phone number -
Maybe I should respect her privacy.
I dialed the number.
"Hi Ethel. It's Mike. I just wanted ask how you were?"
"I'm fine, Mike. I left the hospital in a hurry because they offered to discharge me, and I was anxious to get back home. I'm sorry I didn't say goodbye to you before I left..."
"Ethel, I've been thinking. There are some protein drinks in the health food store that might be good for you. Can I bring you some?..."

The door opened.
Her back was to me -
I followed her sleek figure inside.
The room was dark, and felt like the apartment where my father had lived with his girlfriend.
Boxes were scattered through the hallway - The things inside looked hastily packed.
"Can I offer you something to drink, Mike?"
The refrigerator was stacked with soft drinks and pre-packaged desserts.
"That's okay, Ethel. I brought that protein drink. Would you like to try some?"
She prepared the drink in a blender, then sat with me at the cluttered kitchen table.
"I'm sorry about all the boxes, Mike," she said, looking at me with beguiling eyes. "We just moved into this place.

"I'd been living with my Aunt Belle for a while. She was the same aunt as the one I told you who raised me.

"When I was three years old, I told Momma I wanted to live with Auntie... I just told her I didn't want to live at home anymore, and she said 'Okay.'

"I moved back in with her after my last marriage fell apart.

"I tell you, Mike - That last person I was with - *He was something else!* I'd just gotten out of another relationship when this one came along. *You want to talk about going from the frying pan into the fire!*

"After the wedding, my younger daughter Ivy and I moved into this fella's house. It didn't take me long to figure out what a mistake that was.

"He was constantly asking me questions - Where I was during the day? Where I was going? Accusing me of all kinds of things, *and calling me names.*

"I could handle the verbal abuse - I'd decided a long time ago that I wasn't going to let anything someone said bother me or ruin my day.

"But, when he got started with the physical stuff, I left so fast it made his head spin! *I mean, it literally made his head spin.*

"When I moved in with my aunt, I thought it would be a good thing for us both. She's getting older and I know she needs help.

"But she insisted on treating me just like a child.

"She wanted to know where I was going, what I was doing.

"I wasn't used to that - I was used to doing things in my own way - *And she wasn't going to let me do that.* As long as I was in her house, she was going to make me live by her rules, and that was all there was to it.

"We'd seen this apartment a month before. My older daughter Shoniah had just gotten her real estate license, and showed me this place. I really didn't want it. It's kind of far out and a trip to the medical center. I looked at some places near the medical center, but they were so expensive, Mike - I wasn't going to pay eight hundred dollars for a small apartment.

"But it was just getting so bad at my aunt's house that one day I called Shoniah and said, 'If that place' - this one here - 'was still open, *to take it.'*"

"And, so," she said, moving her feet back and forth. "Here we are..."

"I didn't want to leave the Office of Student Affairs," she said. "I had worked there for twenty years.

"But these new people they brought in - *They were too much.*

"They didn't seem to care, and they weren't polite.

"All they did seem to want to do was talk behind peoples' backs.

"I didn't want to work in that kind of environment, so I gave them my notice.

"I tried to start my own business... Designing emblems for stationery and things... It didn't bring in enough income, though, and I had to find a regular job..."

A look of disgust gripped her features -

"I don't like the way things are going. You turn on the television, all you ever see is crime.

"The Bible says an end of the world is coming. I believed that day is near.

"You look around you - Things aren't getting any better - They're only getting worse.

"What do you think about that, Mike?"

"I suppose I look at life from an evolutionary point of view, Ethel.

"In the beginning, there were unlimited resources, and organisms flourished.

"Now, those resources are dwindling, and if we are to survive as a species, we must find another source of energy - One that is not only recyclable, but, also, self-propagating.

"The only source of energy I know like that is love.

"When you love someone, it grows and snowballs and spreads one to another.

"That's where I think our hope as a species lies..."

"I was reading a book about the evolutionary development of relationships between men and women. The author suggested that early on we were a tree-dwelling species, and mated with whomever we pleased. We were all 'swingers' back then.

"Later, when we left the trees and took to the caves, we had to develop a system whereby the men would be willing to leave for extended periods to go on hunting parties, and perhaps leave one man behind to guard the women. To do this each man took a steady mate, so he would feel there was someone he could come home to. I call these types the 'cavemen'.

"The problem is - Now we have these two patterns of mating ingrained within us, and we're not sure which to choose."

Ethel stared into the distance.

"I don't know, Mike," she said. *"I guess I've always been looking for my soul mate..."*

She went upstairs.

When she reappeared on the stairwell, a child-like aura seemed to radiate from her.

"I guess that one glass of protein drink was probably enough nourishment for the day," she said.

I looked up smiling -

Like a schoolgirl, I thought, who spends ten minutes on her homework, then announces she's ready to go out and play...

I left shortly after.

From the doorway she followed my steps to the car.

"Be careful," she called after me.

She waved as I drove past.

The next day I met Dr. Brand after morning report -

"Dr. Brand, I have some concerns about Ethel. She's taking this nonsteroidal anti-inflammatory drug Baritol. She says it's the only thing taking the edge off the pain, but she's having a lot of pain and bloating, and I'm concerned she's developing an ulcer. I wonder if we shouldn't put her on a prostaglandin agonist like Lytec to counter the Baritol's effects..."

"Mike!" he said curtly. "You've got to remember!..."

He turned away, a deeply etched scowl carved into his features -

"We've got to prepare ourselves."

He stepped to the side -

"What we're watching is something that only takes a down-hill course from here. I've seen it many times with other patients - It's one thing after another until the disease runs its course..."

CHAPTER FOURTEEN

Ethel and I sat at her cluttered kitchen table.

"May I share something with you, Ethel?"

"Yes, Mike."

"I told you that I was ill while I was away in DC, and conventional therapies weren't able to help me. I sought other forms of healing. They did help, and I became trained in using them.

"There's one method in particular I'd like to share with you. It's called bioenergy. Would you like to try it, Ethel?"

"Okay, Mike."

I held out my hand.

"Put your hand over my hand. Try not to touch it. Bioenergy is based on the theory that there's an energetic circulation to the body - One that science hasn't defined yet.

"When the body sustains injury or trauma, blockages in the energetic circulation develop.

"The source of this trauma can be emotional, physical - And, if left untreated, manifest in illness.

"Bioenergy can remove these blockages, and restore the normal flow of energy.

"More than anything else, bioenergy helped me get well..."

"It's still difficult for me to share -

"Unlike drugs, where you can quantify their effects, I don't think you can do that with bioenergy...

"I get afraid people will think I'm trying to mislead them, and that's hard for me because I know how vulnerable sick people are.

"Nevertheless, I can't deny my experience, and, where I think it's appropriate, I extend it to others..."

"Anyway, Ethel. The reason I ask you to place your hand over mine is because, years ago, I discovered I seem to emanate an energy that people can feel - This way I can make bioenergy more tangible, and take away some of the mystery.

"Do you feel anything, Ethel?"

Her eyes were closed and smiling.

"Yes, I do," she said.

"What does it feel like?"

"It feels like puffs of air blowing on my hand."

"What about that?" I said. "You perceive energy the way I do. Most say they feel heat. Others say it feels like tingling or static electricity. When I feel energy, it usually feels like a breeze against my hand.

"Ethel, let's see how sensitive you are. Move your hand back and forth over mine, and see if you don't feel a point where the energy is coming from."

She moved her hand in a circular path.

"It feels like it's coming from your palm."

"Good. That's where most people feel it...

"Now let's try something else - Move your hand up and down my forearm, and see if you can't find another point."

She guided her hand over my arm.

"I feel it there... At about the middle of your arm."

"That's right - That's where people who have a higher acuity feel it. That's great..."

Ethel moved her hand back over my palm. Her eyes closed, the unsure inquisitive smile gracing her features, a captivated glow emanated from her.

"I'm feeling something else now," she said. "It feels like something moving up my arm, and right into my back."

At that moment a painful sensation was happening in my thumb. It had an itchy, tingly, unnatural quality to it -

Like something metallic -

Raw nerve endings stretched over steel.

Why had those words - that image - come to mind?

The intensity of the pain grew worse, as I writhed in my chair to contain it.

"Ethel... I'm feeling something."

"What is it, Mike?"

"It's a sharp pain. Like the muscles in my hand are being stretched beyond their limit..."

"Do you want to stop, Mike?"

Before I could answer she pulled her hand away.
Instantly, the pain disappeared.
Ethel looked away.
*"That's a good way of describing it - What I feel," she said.
"Usually, when the doctors ask me about the pain I'm feeling in my back, I tell them it feels like someone's put me into a vice.*

"But that feeling of 'stretching' - Yeah - that's what it feels like alright. Uh-huh."
"Oh, it's terrible, Ethel! It feels like - pulled any tighter - the muscles will snap and break!"
Ethel nodded.
"Yeah. That's what it feels like..."

I went home, and pulled a book on Reflexology from my shelf. Reflexology was a healing method with its roots in Africa, that correlates specific points on the hands and feet with different parts of the body -
I looked for the place in my thumb where I'd experienced pain at Ethel's.
It mapped to the spine.
Given her back pain, I thought, that makes sense.
But why was *I* feeling it? Why was the pain *she had* registering in me?
I went to my diary, and read through the passages detailing my early experiences at Dr. Amin's clinic -

Monday, September 27, 1993
I am becoming cognizant of a strange phenomenon that is occurring with greater regularity when I work with patients. Rather than derive immediate therapeutic benefit from my efforts, something different happens. I interlink with them, and their symptoms become physically manifest in my own body. I am gripped by a feeling of deep, gnawing chest pain while working with a person whose primary problem is anxiety; or the room begins spinning and I am overcome with dizziness while working with a woman suffering from vertigo and severe nausea related to her pregnancy. Why is this happening? It is as though they'd rather communicate their suffering than attain relief from it...

The next morning I awoke to a feeling of Ethel inside myself.
I saw the two of us together -
Sitting naked on a cloud -
Our eyes closed -

33

She smiling behind me -
A feeling of contentment radiating in all directions...

I got up and looked in the mirror -
"We have to prepare ourselves..."
Let her go alone into that miserable death the illness had in store
for her? -
Or open her to my light?
"Be careful..."
No, I thought.
Life is not miserable when you live it and leave it in love -
Only when you're left alone...

CHAPTER FIFTEEN

I'd been walking to my mailbox when I saw our security guard Chris.

He had been very kind earlier in the month when I'd arrived at my apartment to discover the key the landlord left didn't work -

He contacted a locksmith, then worked well past his shift to help me unload my things...

Chris had extraordinary physical strength -

But what attracted me most was his exuberance, and ability to embrace joy.

"How's it going, Chris?" I said.

"Ah, man. It's not goin' so good... I have this bad pain in my thumb. There all the time... Yeah, constant... I don't know - It's been there a long time... I hurt it playing basketball... Yeah, I'd been going for a slam dunk, and I got my arm caught on the rim or something..."

"Let me take a look?"

I felt for tight muscles -

To my surprise I didn't find any.

"Chris, I'd like to try something else. It's called bioenergy. I'm just going to pass my hand over yours. Is that alright?"

"Yeah, sure, man. Anything you got to do."

I scanned energetically, and felt a vector of energy radiating from his thumb.

I'd been following the strain when a muscle jumped in *my* forearm.

That's funny. I wonder if it's telling me something about Chris?

"Chris, don't ask me why, but I think the pain in your thumb is coming from your forearm.

"Tell me something - If I press on this spot in your arm right here, do you feel anything?"

Instantly, he slumped over and nearly fell to his knees.

"Whatcha doin' man! You're killin' me!..."

"Don't worry, Chris. You'll feel better soon..."

"You're breakin' me down, man!..."

The sun had begun to set -

Looking over at our shadows, one was small and bowed -

The other stood tall and erect...

Gradually, Chris began to straighten -

"Whew, I never experienced anything like that before."

"How does your thumb feel?"

He moved it back and forth.

"It feels better."

"Good. I'll check on you tomorrow."

I went back to my apartment.

For a second time in two days I'd interlinked with someone using bioenergy -

"What is happening?" I thought. "And why now?..."

The next day I went to see him.

"How's your arm, Chris?"

He kept his head down, face turned away from me.

"It's okay."

He had a shame-faced look.

"Let me check it."

"No way, man," he said, pulling his arm away. "I don't know what'chu done - Just squeeze a man's arm, and break him down that way. I ain't never been broken down like that before."

"Chris, let me explain. I wasn't applying pressure there to 'break you down'. I was doing it to treat the muscle.

"You had something called a trigger point - a taut band of muscle that comes about when you injure something.

"When you strain a muscle it often reacts by tightening down - It's like it's saying, 'This guy really hurt me - Now I'm going to make sure he can't do it again!'

"The pain in your thumb probably originated from a problem in your forearm - Something called referred pain.

"When I applied pressure there, I was performing a technique called ischemic compression - It limits the amount of blood that can get to the muscle. Already the blood supply is limited because the muscles are tight - Now the only way the muscle can get enough circulation is to let go of the strain."

I gripped his forearm.
He remained erect.
"You see. The muscle is back to normal. *I can't hurt you now...*"

CHAPTER SIXTEEN

The Board of Medical Examiners had instituted a new licensing exam.

"Most of us take a full month off," a fellow student told me, "and just study before we take it."

I put my remaining rotations on hold, and prepared for the exam.

In between I wrote about my experiences over the last six years.

Ethel was at home now, and no longer working -

"Hey, Ethel, can I read you something?... It's about the clinic where I learned bioenergy..."

Dr. Amin took me in to see my first patient.

"I have a young doctor with me," he said in a soft voice and professional manner to the woman in the examining room. "Would you mind if he came in?"

He motioned me to follow.

The woman inside looked withdrawn and uncomfortable.

He asked her some questions, then directed her to lie on her back, and ran his hand over her abdomen without touching her.

"Feel this," he said, without any explanation.

I approached the woman and passed my hand over her abdomen the way he had.

"Do you feel that?" he said.

Oddly enough I did -

It felt like a breeze, radiating from her abdomen, and blowing against my hand.

"Yes, I do," I said.

"What direction is it going?"

"Wait a minute - You never prepared me for this - What is this?"

"Bioenergy," he said under his breath.

"What's that?"

"It's the body's way of telling you there's a blockage. Energy gets stuck and can't move, so it just collects there. Now feel for what direction it's going."

"How do I do that?"

"Let the energy move your hand in whichever direction it wants to take you."

The energy moved my hand diagonally.

"That's right," he said. "It's a stretch injury. She was wearing a seatbelt when she got hit by another car, and her body got twisted. Now it needs to be corrected."

He took out an oscillating hammer, and applied it to her abdomen until the tension released.

I walked out of the examining room speechless.

In the hallway I looked at Dr. Amin.

He just shrugged his shoulders; his beady eyes unwilling to acknowledge anything out of the ordinary.

For the rest of the day we went from room to room, patient to patient, the same way...

"Mike," Ethel interrupted in excited tones, "when you read what you've written, the words just flow so..."

"There's more, Ethel..."

There could be no substitute for the training I received at Dr. Amin's clinic -

The patients there were in intense pain - most of them suffering for years without reprieve.

An elderly woman brought in by family because of a nagging back -

I casually passed my hand over behind her -

Only to experience what felt like the torrents of a storm blowing from her back.

I looked at her, astonished -

An elderly woman -

Quiet - Stone-faced -

Yet the energy that radiated from her felt like gale-force winds - How could this be?...

Dr. Amin introduced me to a technique called interlink.

The patient lay on the examining table. He suffered from intense low back pain. Dr. Amin instructed me to grasp his ankles. Instantly I became aware of a sensation of tightness in my lower back. I took my hands off - The sensation evaporated. I put them on again - It came back.

But there was something else as well -

A deeper feeling - One of sympathy and concern -

As though a greater connection were being forged between us - An empathic link...

CHAPTER SEVENTEEN

Often Ethel suffered from attacks of severe pain -
"It feels like there are ants crawling all over me..."
She spoke with humor and abandon -
"And I'm shooing them away, but they keep coming back..."
Unlike anything I'd known, or was used to -
"I sure hope they stop crawling on me soon..."
How was it that she could suffer -
And not insist I do the same?...

CHAPTER EIGHTEEN

I phoned Ethel the following day.

"How are you feeling, Ethel?"

"Not too well, Mike. I'm nearly out of my medicines.

"I spoke to the secretary at the Oncology Office yesterday, and she told me Dr. Hood had already written and signed for my medications. But when I sent my younger daughter Ivy to go get them, she wasn't able to find where they were.

"Also, I called the hospital pharmacy, and they told me they didn't have any of the anti-inflammatories I'm taking, and that I'd have to get it from a local pharmacy. But when I called one of the pharmacy out here, they told me a prescription for thirty pills would cost like a hundred dollars..."

"A hundred dollars for thirty pills, Ethel!"

"Yes, Mike. I'd like to use something else less expensive, but the Baritol is the only one that gets rid of the pain. The other medications help, but they don't ever take the pain completely away. Only the Baritol does that.

"I'm going to send Ivy to the hospital again today, and see if she can find the prescriptions this time."

"How much medication do you have left, Ethel?"

"I only have two pills."

"Ethel, I better get it for you. Who knows if Ivy won't run into the same problems again."

"Are you sure, Mike?"

"Yeah. I'll call you from the hospital after I get them..."

I hung up the phone.

"A hundred dollars! Ethel doesn't have that kind of money."

I called the hospital pharmacy.

"We are all out of stock," the pharmacist insisted. "You will have to purchase it at a local pharmacy."

I couldn't believe they would expect their patients to pay that much.

I went to the hospital to ask in person.

"Hi, I called earlier about the Baritol earlier. Would you mind if I asked you to look for it again?"

"Wait here," the pharmacist said. "I'll look for it."

He came back a few minutes later.

"We have it. But it's a non-formulary medication. You will need to get a special request, and have it signed by a physician."

I went to the Oncology Office.

Dr. Hood looked up from the group of students he was with.

"Is there something, Mike?"

"Yeah. Ethel needs some Baritol. Would you mind signing for it?"

"Sure, Mike." He hurriedly took the prescription. "I also prescribed Morphine sulfate for her. It's fast acting and will relieve intense breakthrough pain. A special triplicate form is required for narcotics like morphine. I wrote for it yesterday. You'll find it posted at the Oncology clinic..."

At the Oncology clinic there were two nurses.

"Hi, I'm looking for a prescription for Ms. Ethel James."

They looked at me with bored, blank expressions.

"Dr. Hood said it was posted somewhere," I said.

Celia glanced over at Karen with a knowing look, then lifted a hand in the other direction and tapped her long fingernails on the bulletin board where a prescription was pinned.

I took the prescription.

"Thank you."

Their eyes followed me as I left the room...

On the way to the pharmacy, though, I noticed the prescription wasn't signed -

I'm going to have to find Dr. Hood again.

I went back to the Oncology Office.

"Do you have something for me, Mike?" Dr. Hood said.

"Yeah, Dr. Hood. The prescription for morphine needs to be signed."

"Oh. Okay..."

I stood in line at the pharmacy.

"This prescription for morphine is not correct," the pharmacist said. "It is written for 10 milligrams. We do not carry that dose. You will have to get a new prescription."

I went back to the Oncology Office -

This time Dr. Hood and his team were no longer there.

"They're probably on rounds," the secretary said.

I went from floor to floor looking.

"God, do other people have this much trouble?"

I found him on the D wing of the fifth floor.

"What's up, Mike?"

"The pharmacy doesn't have a 10 milligram dose. Only 30 or 60 milligrams."

"Oh."

He wrote for the smaller dose...

"This correction is illegible!" the pharmacist insisted. "We cannot honor it!"

"But I've just seen Dr. Hood," I said. "I had to hunt him down all over the hospital. *He initialed the dose change.*

"Look, I'm getting this for a patient, who's out of her pain medications. If she doesn't get her medicine soon, it's gonna send her into a pain crisis.

"Now I'm going to re-write the dose change, and I'll initial it as well."

I pushed it back through the opening in the window.

He gave me a long, careful look through the bulletproof glass.

"Alright," he said. "It will take about an hour for us to fill this prescription. You can have a seat over there..."

An hour later another pharmacist was behind the counter.

"Here is the prescription," she said, opening a chute under the counter and sliding me a brown paper bag.

I checked the medications.

"Wait a minute!" I said. "This is the wrong form of morphine. It's continuous release... That won't cover breakthrough. She needs straight morphine - It was written for on the prescription..."

The pharmacist took the medications and ran to her supervisor.

The supervisor pushed his way to the window.

"What's the matter here?!" he said.

"I was given the wrong medication."

He examined the prescription.

"You will have to wait. There are several forms that have to be completed when errors like these come up..."

Mid afternoon I called Ethel with the correct medications.
"How are you doing, Ethel?"
"Not so good, Mike. The pain is pretty bad."
"I'll be right over."
I raced to her apartment -
All the time asking myself, *"What do other people do?..."*

I arrived at Ethel's, and sat with her as she took the morphine.
"The medications are working," she said. "I don't feel as bad now."
"Oh, thank God," I said...

CHAPTER NINETEEN

Ethel and I were sitting at her kitchen table when I heard a 'pop' from upstairs, and the sound of heavy footsteps overhead.

Ethel curled up in her chair, cringing.

"That's Matthew," she said under her breath.

Her eyes looked vigilant and hyper-alert.

"He's okay."

A handsome African American man appeared at the top of the stairs.

"H-e-l-l-o," he said in a deep, resonant, reassuring tone, as he made his way down the stairs.

He was large and robust -

But the way he moved - his content belly leading the way - had the aura of a happy little boy, and immediately endeared me -

"Hi, I'm Mike," I said, shaking his hand.

"Y-e-a-h. Nice - to - meet - you. I've - heard - a - lot - about - you..."

Then, as suddenly as he'd appeared, he left through the front.

Ethel remained hunched, eyes following him.

"Matthew and I have been friends since childhood," she said in a detached, wary tone. *"When I was admitted to the hospital, I wrote his name in the box for 'Significant other.'*

"He has a difficult time with illness. He didn't come to see me..."

Ethel went to the kitchen.

"Mike, would you like to stay for dinner. I'd like to make some steak, but I'm worried that it might not sit well with your stomach, being that you're mostly vegetarian."

"Oh, I'd like to have some meat, Ethel. I think my muscles are craving it..."

She cooked the steaks.

"Here, Mike," she said, handing me a plate. "I hope you enjoy it."

We sat at the cluttered table.

"Mmm. This is really good, Ethel."

"I'm glad you like it, Mike."

"Yeah, it's really good. Mmm. Mmm."

Then, I caught myself.

"Oh, Ethel, I'm sorry. Here I am still making 'mmm' sounds."

"That's alright, Mike. You say 'mmm' all you like."

"You won't send me to my room, Ethel?"

"No, Mike." She looked at me intently. "I'm happy you're enjoying your food..."

At home it wasn't long before a cocoon of scintillating energy enveloped me.

I lay in bed -

One-by-one, the trigger points in my body spontaneously untangled and released -

It was as though some invisible energetic hands were working on me -

Delicately effecting a release in one muscle, then moving to the next...

CHAPTER TWENTY

I was making my way to the Claude Ray when I looked up and saw the tall, lanky figure of Dr. Brand gliding towards me.

"How are you doing, Mike?" he said in a gentle, heart-felt tone, *shaking my hand. "How is Ms. James?"*

"She's alright. I saw her the other day."

"Oh, yeah... Where does she live?"

"South of town. Near Airport and Main Street."

He frowned and nodded.

"Not bad. Not too long a ride from the medical center."

"I'm heading to the medical school," he said. "I'm teaching this course in Mechanisms and Management of Disease. They have a review every Monday at noon."

"I'll walk with you."

We took a short cut through the corridors of the old Claude Ray Hospital.

"Pancreatic cancer is a terrible disease," he said. "It's not like a lot of other cancers where you can point to a definite cause. At least with lung cancer you can say it's because the person smoked. With pancreatic you can't do that."

I hesitated.

"By coincidence, my anatomy professor also died of pancreatic cancer," I said. "I'd been the medical student assigned to take care of him when he came to the hospital. I actually wrote a short story about it..."

"Oh, I enjoy writing, too. I'd like to write a novel. I have the beginning - 'As the man in the bed lay dying he thought he had led a happy life.'" He laughed irrepressibly. "A beginning like that I thought would engage the reader... I don't have the rest yet... Mostly I write Spanish poetry these days...

"I'd like to read your story, though..."

I slipped a copy of Rebirth under his door the next day -

In a darkened room he lay; his piercing gaze fixed on the bare white-washed wall in front of him; never leaving their singular focus... This only marred by the brief lapses in concentration provoked by the annoying short white-jacketed figure standing adjacent to him.

The short white-jacketed figure was taking notes; he wore an expression of deep contemplation - the source of which not so much the result of meticulous inspection as the product of a preposterous feeling that grips one faced with pursuing a futile endeavor.

The disease that had so ravaged the patient's body had only been recognized a week before. He had been at a chili cook-off when he noticed an uncomfortable feeling of fullness. Following a check-up and several subsequent tests, he'd been given at best a few months to live.

A respected professor, well loved by his students - Affable, considered by many a kindred spirit. To the short white-jacketed figure (note-pad in hand) he was none of these; to the man in the bed these feelings were mutual...

A year ago in the anatomy laboratory -

"The physician does have a stake in society," he told his classmates. "By his mere position he is in-trusted with the care and responsibility for others; he must put the good of the community first, go where he is called, sacrifice when need be, and place the welfare of others ahead of his own..."

Then, from behind, the resounding bellow -

"What is the source of this man's guilt?"

His classmates broke out in laughter. Looking around he saw the wily professor, smiling, before cheerfully making his way to the next tank...

The hateful examination progressed. Meaningless palpations, percussions, measurements. During rounds "Let me go" his only request. No visitors permitted; all well-wishers turned away. Students lined the halls, come to offer their last respects. Now he was the one student permitted in his presence - And he loathed him.

"Put your arms in front of you and hold them still." The simple command came out like all the others - But, really, he had to tense his body and force the words through his lips, as what followed was

their least favorite part of the exam, and a site that always unnerved him.

The professor dutifully and disdainfully complied; his severe gaze never leaving him. Against the weight of massive ascites, he lifted himself into a half-seated position, then raised his arms - palms up, fingers extended.

Within an instant, his arms fell. He pulled them back - They fell again. Over and over - As though some invisible support they'd been resting on had been pulled from underneath him.

Straining, the man in the bed summoned the force of his will. But it was no use, as the spectacle only repeated itself.

The short white-jacketed figure looked on, fascinated and appalled and having hard time collecting himself.

"That's enough," he cried.

The professor dropped his arms. Relief quickly replaced by disgust; smoldering anger permeating his features, as he kept his gaze averted, and meanly stared at the wall in front of him.

"That's all." He left the room...

A review of the physical and laboratory findings suggested he would die some time during the night. There was nothing to be done; no resuscitation orders; no monitoring or supportive care. He wanted to be there. Not for love; only the experience.

The door remained shut. No visitors permitted. No requests. His orders to be left alone.

The short white-jacketed figure lumbered into the nursing station. He'd been on call the night before. He slouched into a chair, his body conforming to its contours. Resting his head on his hand, he leaned against the armrest...

The cave was dark. A vaporous mist rose from its bowels, and an ill red-tinged glow enveloped him. A feeling of cold detachment dominated his senses as he plodded deeper, driven by some unknowable urge to venture forth.

Then, he felt another presence. Turning, he saw a hillside - Pitched against a clear blue sky. A group of hikers - healthy and robust - made their way along a trail of trees and green shrubs. His heart elated, he looked back and saw them stopped and smiling.

"Come on up," the leader motioned.

In that moment he could plainly see himself between the hillside and the abyss. He turned and stared into the darkness - Saw the mist and red-tinged glow. The feeling of detachment resurfaced and the maniacal curiosity to know what lay beyond. Feet planted he looked into the darkness. Then, in an effortless gesture, stepped forward - Into the light...

He awoke to a strange sensation. His head cocked over his hand, he felt his pulse under his neck. I'm alive, he thought and wondered. I'm alive.

Shaking off the vestiges of sleep, he got to his feet, and with deliberate, heavy steps made his way to his professor's room. Gently, quietly, he pushed at the door. Rays of light streamed into the room. From the doorway, he looked in. His chest didn't move. Was this it? he thought. Was this the end?

Suddenly, he inhaled with violent force - A crashing sound that sent Michael reeling back, and nearly threw Dr. Woodley from the bed. "Who's there?" he cried out in a startled voice. Michael ran to his side.

"It's me, Dr. Woodley. I'm sorry... I'm sorry I disturbed you...."
"No... It's alright."
The words were kind and left him shaken.
"Can I get you anything?"
"No... no... I'm okay."
That same sweetness, and he trembled as he rose.
Something inside wanted to hold on to life - Something else told him it was alright.
"Good-night, then."
"Good-night." And his words rose and filled the room.
Turning, he walked to the door.
Then, midway there, a rush of cool air blew at his back.
The urgency resurfaced - But this time he didn't look 'round.
Still possessed by the alien sweetness of the dying man's parting words, he left the room...

I arrived early at Morbidity and Mortality conference on Friday - Dr. Brand was sitting in the middle of the room.
"I read your story," he said. "Was that really something that happened?"
"Yes."
"Did he actually say that to you?... About the guilt?"
"'What is the source of this man's guilt?' Yes, I'll always remember."
"What made him say something like that to you?!"
"I suppose he understood me."
"You think that's it?!"

"I don't know - Maybe there was something else, too. He was a hard man."

"When was this?"

"1991. Right after I left your service."

"And he wouldn't take any visitors?... What was that about?"

"I don't know. They lined the hallways. I watched them sit against the walls of the corridors all day. Some classmates I really liked and respected. He wouldn't see them."

"Why was that?"

"I don't think he thought they really knew him. I mean, on the one hand, he was a born-again Christian; on the other, he was homosexual..."

"You see! Those are things that need to be in your story. Right now you have a lot there, but it needs to be developed. The characters are interesting - the plot. It's too cryptic, though. I know you so I can kind of read between the lines and fill-in the details, but I think you could really expand this."

"As a matter of fact, after I gave it to you, I re-wrote it - And made it even more cryptic. I want the reader to make up his or her own mind, and not be swayed by what I think."

"Yeah, I have the same feelings when I write - 'Am I being judgmental?'

"But the things like you just told me - They have a place there..."

CHAPTER TWENTY-ONE

"Whenever I lay on my right side," Ethel said, "it feels like my insides are shifting, and piling up on top of each other.

"I've told this to many of the doctors who I spoke to, but none of them were able to offer an explanation."

"I wonder if it would respond to the things I do, Ethel," I said. "Would you like me to come over and try?"

"Not today, Mike," she said. "Earlier in the morning I decided I wanted to devote the day to rest. I haven't had a strict day of rest in almost a week, and it's been six days since I started the cancer medication. Already I'm losing some of my hair, and I can't taste my food the way I used to.

"Shoniah came over this weekend, and brought Sammy. She had some things she had to do, so I told her to leave the baby with me.

"He's so curious, Mike! He just always wants to know everything that's going on!

"But he's one of those children who fight sleep... You know, they're so interested in what's going on around them that they don't want to take naps.

"I found a way to coax him to sleep, though... I take him in bed with me, and gently rub his back - That way he knows there's someone there, and doesn't feel like he's missing as much..."

Hanging up the phone, waves of energy descended over me.
I lay in bed, drifting off to sleep -
Wishing she were with me...

CHAPTER TWENTY-TWO

"I'm still having these stomach problems, Mike," Ethel said. "I have an appointment at the medicine clinic today. I hope they can tell me something."

"Ethel, would you mind if I went with you? I'd like to see what they say..."

That afternoon I sat waiting for Ethel on the second floor of the Claude Ray.

I'd been reading a review book when I saw her enter the corridor.

Her movements were as fluid and effortless as ever -

But at the reception area she bent steeply, and supported herself against the counter.

"Hi, Ethel. How are you doing?"

"Oh, fine, Mike. My daughter drove me... She's still in the car finishing some food she bought at Libby's on the way over here. I wanted to check on my lab results, but the woman at the front says she doesn't have them."

"I'll get them for you, Ethel."

I went to the ward and printed the reports.

When I came back, Ethel was in a crowded holding area - And my eyes were drawn to a shy, vulnerable-looking young woman sitting a few chairs down from her.

"Mike, I want you to meet my daughter Shoniah."

Ethel had spoken of Shoniah often -

"She's a lot like you, Mike," she'd said. "She has so many talents and interests.

"But it worries me because I think it's hard for her to do just one thing..."

Ethel kept several photos of Shoniah on her mantelpiece -

Looking at them I saw a demure young woman, who, I surmised, was mean-spirited.

Now, the young woman who sat before me appeared sweet and good-natured -

Just as Ethel had described her...

It was cold in the holding area, and I went to the wards to find some blankets.

"Ethel, why don't you cover yourself with these."

She wrapped herself in the blankets - Then stared at something behind me, as though waiting for it to pass.

I looked over my shoulder -

A janitor was pushing his cart -

"What'chu 'fraid of?" he directed at Ethel. "Somebody lookin' at you? Shit! Don't need t' worry 'bout that - Ever'body else do it!"

Ethel and I exchanged smiles. Then she laid her head down and closed her eyes; the embarrassed inquisitive expression still gracing her features...

Ethel's name was called, and she, Shoniah and I went into the examining room.

A resident entered -

"So, how are you doing?" he said.

Although pleasant, he had the look of a person who was only half there.

"Not so good," Ethel responded. "I'm having problems with my stomach. It feels like there's a lot of air there - And the intestines feel like they're shifting..."

"'Air there,'" he repeated. "'Shifting'..."

"And I've developed these patchy white spots under my tongue..."

"'Patchy white spots'..."

"What do you think they are?" she asked.

"It's probably normal," he responded gruffly.

He performed a brief examination, and prepared to leave.

"I'm sorry I got you into trouble that one time with Dr. Brand," Ethel remarked after him.

"Oh!" he said, and, for the first time, came out of his fog. "That's alright."

He left the room.

Ethel turned to me -

"The time I'd been seen in clinic by Dr. Brand, he was the first one to examine me.

"When I was admitted to the hospital, I saw him again, and said hello.

"But he didn't recognize me, or remember who I was.

"I said, 'You examined me the other day with Dr. Brand.'

"'No, I didn't, lady,' he says. 'I don't know you.'

"When Dr. Brand came in, he says to him, 'You don't remember, Ms. James?!'

"And then he said a few more things..."

The resident came back to the room -

"We're going to prescribe you mycelex," he announced.

"What is that for?" Ethel said.

"The thrush in your mouth."

"Is that what these white patches are under my tongue?..."

"Yes!" he interrupted. "It's thrush!..."

He left, and the oncology nurse Karen came in -

She needed to collect some blood samples, and stuck Ethel several times without success.

Finally, she found a vein -

But lost it mid-collection.

"I'm sorry I'm such a difficult stick," Ethel told Karen, smiling. "Maybe, it was my fault because I opened my hand at the time the blood stopped flowing."

She had to start over.

"Maybe, we should go to the blood drawing station," I said.

"No, Mike," Ethel responded. "We don't want to have to go all the way over there. You go ahead Karen..."

Karen found a vein, and collected the sample.

Ethel left the room to give a urine specimen, leaving Shoniah and I alone.

"I'm glad she gets to eat now," she said.

"'Gets to'?!" I responded. "You mean 'Can eat now'?!"

"'Can' - 'Gets to' - It's *better.*"

She smiled.

I looked away, annoyed.

"Those protein drinks seem really good," she said.

"Yes. I think they help her a lot."

"Yeah, I think I should get some..."

Celia, the other oncology nurse, sat behind the front desk.

"Prescriptions!" She slammed them on the counter. "Blood drawings!" Slam. "CT exams!" Slam. "Follow-up appointments!..."

Ethel was bent over the desk -

"If I have a problem," she said, "will it be alright for me to call the clinic?"

Celia looked up at her with a bored expression.

"Why, what do you mean?" she said in a slow, deliberately condescending tone of voice.

"I mean, if I get into some trouble - with the pain or whatever - will there be someone here who I can call and talk to about coming in or scheduling an immediate appointment?"

"The clinic is usually full," she responded, "and there probably wouldn't be room to schedule an appointment for you."

The other day Ethel told me that one of the nurses had belittled her -

"'Just because you knew Dr. Hood when he was a medical student,' she said, 'doesn't mean you should expect special treatment.'"

Celia looked at me -

"If something urgent should arise," she said, "you could go to the emergency center."

"This is my private card," she added. "If anything should happen, you can call me at this number..."

I escorted Ethel to the pharmacy, then downstairs and outside where Shoniah was waiting in the car.

"Mike, do you need a lift?" Ethel asked.

They drove me to the parking lot.

I waved as they drove off...

That evening energy penetrated the top of my head, and flowed into my legs.

My body began to tremble -

What is happening? I thought.

I turned over in bed.

It felt like the very core of my being was shaking -

Unearthing itself, and burrowing its way to the surface...

I called Ethel the next morning.

"I wasn't able to sleep at all last night," she said. "I kept on thinking about that clinic appointment yesterday.

"I felt so disappointed, Mike. The resident didn't answer any of my questions."

"I know, Ethel. It was all I could do to keep from saying anything!

"But that's the way it is in conventional medicine - They don't know how to deal with subacute illness. 'Come back when you're really sick, and you have something for us to cut on!' - Why do you think I'm leaving?..."

CHAPTER TWENTY-THREE

"I just haven't been able to get a handle on the pain this week," Ethel said. "I don't know what it is.

"Maybe, it's because I just did too many things, with going to the doctor's appointment all day and all - then spending the next day at social security. I know I shouldn't do that, but sometimes I just push myself."

She put her head down and laughed.

"I don't know why this pain won't go away. Maybe it's because I strained myself carrying the baby. I hate to think I'm getting worse, and not getting better. I try to keep a positive mind."

I held out my hand.

As soon as she put hers over it, a thick cloud of energy crept up my arm. My airways became constricted, as though I were being gripped by the throat. My heart began to race, and I had the feeling that at any moment I would burst.

This is fear, I thought. I must be tapping into Ethel.

But when I looked across at her, her eyes were closed , expression peaceful.

Perhaps her feelings are moving through me.

I opened myself as much as I could -

"What are you feeling, Ethel?"

"Relaxed!" she said. "It's like the pain is moving out and I get really comfortable.

"It's strange, though, because as soon as that happens, I begin feeling the pain somewhere else."

I got up, and scanned her energetically.

A strain radiated from her forehead, and I followed it until it released -

This led to a large outpouring of energy all over her body - Like a waterfall flowing to the ground.

Returning to my chair, I felt immersed in energy -

"I'd like to work on you some more," I said. "But it feels like the energy is holding me here."

"Maybe it was all those months of nausea and vomiting that are affecting me?" she said. "Or the damage to the spleen? Maybe it's because of the blockages in those vessels? Or perhaps something to do with that liver biopsy?"

A feeling of joy and surrender swept over me -

It's all over now, I thought.

"Ethel," I said, "let's see if the pain in your back isn't related to the muscles of your spine..."

There had always been a reason not to examine her -

I didn't want her to feel uncomfortable -

If it were cancer-related, there was nothing I could do.

Now, as I lay my hands there, I could feel the taut muscles -

And waves of sadness traveled through me that I hadn't looked earlier...

I gently applied pressure -

Right under my fingertips the muscles trembled and released.

"How do you feel now, Ethel?"

"My back feels better," she said, "but now I have this pain in my stomach."

I massaged her abdomen until the muscles relaxed.

"Thank you, Mike. I'm feeling much better now."

I sat back at the table.

"I guess that's just the way it going to happen," she said. "It will just come back and forth."

"No, Ethel, it's not like that. It's like peeling away the layers of an onion - You get beyond one layer, then you go to the next..."

"Until you reach its core," she said...

She smiled now, and lifted her head as she spoke.

Earlier in the day she'd pressed her hand to mine when I'd offered bioenergy -

"No," I'd said. "Over my hand."

"Oh," she smiled. "No touching ..."

CHAPTER TWENTY-FOUR

When I got home I called Ethel to make sure she was still okay.

"Oh, I'm feeling much better," she said. "Matthew is over now, and the two of us are talking."

I was afraid my call might upset him, and quickly got off.

It was a couple days before I called again...

"I'm not doing too good, Mike... Nothing is controlling the pain, and it hasn't gone away since you came over last...

"The days seem to go on so long. When was it that you were here last... Saturday? You see, for some reason I thought it was Thursday.

"My back is hurting, and also my stomach, and I can't seem to get any relief from either. I don't know whether it's because of the tumor, or from the medicines they're giving me."

"Would you like me to come over, Ethel, and see what we can do?"

"Do you think it will do any good, Mike?"

"I don't know, Ethel. But I'd like to try..."

At her kitchen table I held out my hand; she put hers over it and, smiling, closed her eyes.

Instantly, the energy enclosed around my fingers, and pulled me towards her.

I knelt in front of her.

"Ethel, if it's okay, lean forward on your chair. I'm going to reach my arms around you, and massage your back."

Her body draped over my shoulder I probed her muscles until the knots released.

I got up and walked behind her.

"Ethel, this time I'm going to reach my arms around your sides, and gently massage your stomach."

Rubbing in a clockwise motion, the muscles began to relax.

As I went deeper, I felt something hard under my fingertips.

Was this the tumor? I thought. Am I doing harm?

The thought of causing cancer cells to release and spread filled me with apprehension.

No, I thought. It doesn't work like that -

Millions of cells break off tumors everyday -

The reason that some take root in other parts of the body is mostly because they evade the immune system -

Focus on opening the area, and facilitating the circulation there.

I continued to massage her.

Resting my head against her back, I listened to her breath.

I thought about the area I was massaging -

The solar plexus.

I thought about the many emotional traumas Ethel had been through -

Her last marriage - The failed business venture - The difficulties with her aunt.

I love you, Ethel.

Suddenly, the muscles of her abdomen went limp, and her whole body slumped forward on the table...

"What happened, Mike?" she said, lifting her head.

"You fell asleep, Ethel."

"I did?" she said. "I've never done that before."

"I think your body needed it..."

That evening waves of energy descended over me -

They spread like a waterfall spilling over the left side of my head.

My left leg began to pulsate, as trigger points twitched, then spontaneously released.

"Sometimes," Ethel had said earlier, "I think, 'I wish that I could just be pulled at - To stretch these tight muscles... Like someone would just put me on a rack or something. Or, maybe, two people could just get on either side, and pull me at both ends...'"

Thoughts of holding her - Pulling at her sleek figure - Feeling her body give way...

CHAPTER TWENTY-FIVE

Wednesday, October 1, 1997

It was raining when I arrived at Ethel's -
I rang the doorbell.
Where is she?! I thought. I'm not that early!
Just as I was about to go back to my car, I heard a click at the door.

"Was that you, Mike?" Ethel said. "I was in the shower. I thought I heard something. Were you out there long?..."

She led me inside.

There were groceries strewn on the floor from the entranceway to the kitchen.

"What's with the groceries, Ethel?"

"Oh, I went to the store, but I was in pretty severe pain when I got back, so I asked the kids to bring them in for me."

And this is how they leave them for you?!

"Here are your medications, Ethel."

"Oh, thank you, Mike. I've had a really disappointing day. I've been calling Dr. Hood about becoming a private patient, and he won't return my phone calls.

"Then, I called the people at St. Joseph's to find out if the medicine clinic at Claude Ray had faxed them the results of the blood tests, and the nurse there said that not only hadn't they received them, but that they might have to take me off their protocol because of the problems I've been having.

"So I decided that I was going to call the nurses at the Oncology clinic to tell them about this - And do you know what they told me,

Mike? - 'Oh, Mrs. James. To what do we owe the unexpected pleasure of this phone call.'"

"Ethel, I hate to tell you this, but, in many ways, your health is completely in your hands.

"You have to let people help you. I mean, look at this place - The kids bring in the groceries, but don't put them away - Even when they know how difficult it is for you! You have to ask for help, Ethel. Perhaps for the first time in your life - You have to give up some of your independence and let others help you.

"People love you, Ethel. You've accumulated a lot of brownie points. It's time to cash in your chips. You can. Others will be better for it."

"I know," she said, "but I hate to ask people for things."

"Ethel, did I ever tell you about the time I got so tired of asking people for help I nearly entered a fast for a few days?... The pain in my leg had gotten so bad I couldn't drive the car. The mere thought of it sent shivers down my spine. I'd been asking people in my program to get food for me when they went to the market. This had gone on for a month, and it was getting old. I ran out of food, and decided I would just fast for a few days..."

"And this wasn't something you were doing because you thought it would be good for you?" she interrupted.

"Oh, no, Ethel. Going without food was the last thing my body needed. But I just couldn't bear to ask for one more thing.

"I turned out the light, and decided I was just going to sleep through the next three days.

"Then, the phone rang - It was a friend of mine - Said she was going shopping - Asked if I needed anything.

"I cried.

"I'd been working on a vaccine for cancer - I was looking to do something for the millions -

"Yet, at that moment, what mattered to me most was a little bit of food, and someone who cared enough to call."

"I think a lot of people have a problem with me being sick," she said. "My daughter Ivy in particular. She just wants to go about like everything's alright - Like Mommie's there to take care of her like before."

"It can't be that way anymore, Ethel. Now you're the one who needs help..."

It was getting late, and I was ready to go home -

"Ethel, can I help you put this stuff away? Some of it looks kind of heavy."

"That's okay, Mike. If I have a problem, I can get Matthew to do it."

I stood frozen.

"Matthew's here?!"

I thought about standing in the rain.

"He must sleep sound!" I said, directing my voice upwards.

"He does!" she said. "You know, he does that electrical work. That's some important work. You make one mistake, and you can really cause some trouble. I think it's the intellectual part of it that really makes you tired, though..."

Matthew groaned from the bedroom.

Lazy bastard! I thought. What do you see in him!

"Even in my job," she continued. "They think that it's easy because you're sitting at a desk all day. But some of the personalities you come in contact with and have to deal with, and believe me you feel tired at the end of the day..."

She was smiling, and looking at me with all that light.

"Don't be angry with me, Mike," she seemed to be saying. "Don't be upset. Don't leave."

But I couldn't shake my hurt expression, and didn't want to be seen.

"I better go," I said...

I kept my gaze fixed ahead as I drove past.

Out of the corner of my eye I saw her silhouette -

Standing in the doorway...

At home I sat at my desk and tried to study.

It wasn't fair, I thought. Everything I do for her. And still she spends all her time with this guy who does nothing?!

I lay in bed and tried to sleep.

Unlike all the other times I'd come home from being with her, there were no sensations of energy...

On the wards I was attending a pretty young woman.

I asked if she kept a gun in her purse.

She did, and took it out for me.

I bent low and kissed her in plain view of the other doctors.

Then I took a gun from my bag, and pointed it at her -

There was a man sitting next to her. I told him to move off.

"You know what to do," I said.

She gestured to slide off her pants -

Then, took her gun, and shot me in the chest.

My muscles shuddered, and I was thrown to the ground.

"Good," I said.
I remained lying there -
Wondering whether I had sustained a flesh wound, or if the bullet had pierced my lung -
If I should go on living -
Or die?...

I awoke, and thought of Ethel.
It wasn't fair to want her to live a certain way.
Sure, I wanted more - And was jealous of Matthew *who did!*
But, in the end, love would find me anywhere.
Don't do this, Mike. Don't leave ...

CHAPTER TWENTY-SIX

I had an unused airline ticket, and decided to fly back to the east coast.

I called my friend Al Lee, and made plans to visit.

"So, what about this woman you wrote about in your letter?" he said.

"It's hard to explain Al. It's like all of my thoughts about life and the Universe go from an intellectual exercise to something real when I'm with her...

"Al, there are many times when I'm with Ethel that I'm reminded of you and Jun-li."

"Yes." His voice trailed off. "Did I ever tell you about what happened at Master Shou's temple when Jun-li died?...

"When Jun-li initiated into Chi Gong, me and the other assistants worked on her. We formed a circle around her, and transferred our energy to her, one-by-one.

"When it was my turn, I feel a real connection with her.

"Later, after the practice, she came up to me and told me that when other people worked on her she didn't feel anything - Like they were just doing it to be helpful, but there wasn't much there.

"But with me, she said she could really feel something...

"The next day I took her to the Great Falls Park, near my house. It was so beautiful. We sat on the rocks and looked at the falls.

"She turned to me and said this would probably be the last time she'd ever be there and wouldn't see it again.

"I held her - She cried for a long time. She talked about the things she was going to miss - Her life - Her family - Her children - And just to be that close to another person was very special for me..."

A year ago standing outside the Rockville Metro -
Al pulled up in his car.

"Mike," he said, full of excitement. "Don introduced me to a cousin who has pancreatic cancer, and I feel a real connection with her..."

We sped through Potomac, all the time Al talking about his experience with Jun-li.

Something about the way he spoke - his hope and optimism - gave me the intuitive feeling that he truly could help this woman...

In the darkened gymnasium a woman sat in the center of the floor.

Several senior members circled around her.

She was frail and emaciated -

I couldn't perceive her breathing...

"We have two new members," Don Ko announced after practice. "Brad and Jun-li. They are coming from upstate New York. Jun-li is staying with Joanne and me. Brad has to go back tonight."

Don turned to Brad.

"Is there anything you'd like to say to the group before you go, Brad?"

Unlike the rest of us who'd been sitting in a circle, Brad was standing off to the side.

He wore a sweatshirt that looked a couple of sizes too big, and hung off him like a hand-me-down from an older sibling.

"No," he said, in a deliberately hurtful tone...

Don called a few days later.

"Jun-li has some questions," he said. "We thought because of your medical background you might be able to answer them..."

On Sunday I went to his home -

Jun-li was sitting on the couch - Nearly swallowed by its well-cushioned pillows.

"So," she said. "You wanted to tell me something."

In the faint light that filtered through the windows I thought the tiny woman who sat before me looked hard and commandeering.

"Sure," I said -

But, really, I was thinking, *"No. I'm here because Don asked me. I don't want to tell you anything."*

There was a certain meanness about her - A feeling of entitlement.

She struck me as the kind of person not unwilling to walk over others to get what she wanted.

"Yes, she's a very driven person," Al told me later. "She told me so herself. She said she and her husband have worked very hard to get to where they are, and like to have things their own way.

"But some people are like that, Mike. I don't hold that against her..."

I talked about my experience -
The cancer vaccine, and my illness;
Experimental protocols, and Chi Gong.

"So, what do you think?" she said.

"I think in Al Lee, you've found the person who could help you most."

She looked to the side, and, for the first time, her features softened.

"My husband wants me to come home. He says he's found a doctor who is willing to treat me."

Then, her features paled, as though a shroud had been pulled over her.

"I don't want to go. But he is my husband. He tells me he made sacrifices for me - *That I owe him..."*

Later in the week Don called again.

"Jun-li's husband wants to take her back to New York, and Jun-li is very upset and says she doesn't want to go.

"Brad is a chemist. Perhaps, because you are a researcher, you can talk to him..."

I called him that evening.

"I believe in all that!" he said. "If I wanted to, I could take her to the best Chi Gong masters in mainland China!

"But I've been surfing the Web, and found a couple of experimental protocols that combine oriental herbal remedies with chemotherapy, and they sound promising!..."

He went on for a long time -
I listened feeling there was little I could say.

"Do you agree with me?!" he demanded.

I hesitated.

"I agree with everything you've said.

"Still, I can't help but feel that, just by serendipity, in Al Lee you've found the person who can help your wife most."

"But the experimental protocols!" he pleaded. "They might work, right?!"

"Yeah, sure," I said. "I mean, *time will tell.*"

He gasped and broke off, then sobbed for a long time.

"Okay," he said. "I'll let her stay another week."

His voice was calm, and out of breath.

"But after that," he said, resuming his former tone, "I'm coming down to see her, and I don't care what any of you say!..."

"Her husband came," Al said, "and took her away a week later.

"I could understand his reasons - She didn't have a lot of time left, and he wanted her to spend it with the children.

"Shortly after they started her on chemotherapy, her liver stopped working.

"I called and called her - But each time her husband answered, and told me Jun-li couldn't come to the phone - She was too weak.

"I was at Master Shou's house in California when we got the news Jun-li died.

"Master Shou told us to make a circle and let the thought of Jun-li enter our minds.

"I was doing this, when, all of a sudden, this surge of electricity entered my body through my crown chakra.

"I could hear Jun-li's voice inside me -

"Saying she was alright - And she was happy - And things were okay...

"I burst out sobbing - Tears rolling down my face -

"I couldn't stop it - I rolled on the floor, back and forth...

"The others gathered around me. 'What is wrong with Al?' I heard them saying. 'Why is he crying? He must feel really bad.'

"But I was happy. I was happy that she was okay - That she was fine..."

He broke off.

"After that experience, I know there is more than this world...

"I am not afraid of death - It is just another part of life. And the things that happen to people are not by accident - There was a reason I should meet Jun-li...

"Still, I do feel lonely, though..."

CHAPTER TWENTY-SEVEN

"Ethel, I wrote a short piece about Dr. Brand and me. Would you like to hear it?... I call it Beloved."

The short white-jacketed figure returned after a six-year hiatus. He entered the service of his cherished mentor in the place that held for him the most meaning.

His mentor made a deliberate detour during rounds. The patient in the distant corner had a special finding. With the diaphragm of the stethoscope securely pressed against the patient's abdomen he removed the ear-piece.

"Taken a listen to this."

He'd been in the back of the room furthest from the patient and hadn't the slightest knowledge what the detour had been about. A scintillating feeling took hold as he eagerly moved forward.

Reaching the side of the bed adjacent to his mentor, he happily took the ear-piece, and pressed them into his own ears.

"You hear that?"

Cool and unpretentious was his mentor's voice. In this man he'd found an attending with whom he experienced a feeling of kinship. He had had a difficult time on the wards. Different from the others, he had never made any attempt at concealing his deficiencies. Long before he'd made up his mind that the only way to mend his inadequacies was to keep them in plain view - and gamesmanship was never part of the agenda.. But despite his good intentions, his openness was not appreciated; in an environment where most had trained in a kind of old school that taught concealing ones faults, he was foreign, and his fragile frame bore the scars of many a poignant experience.

This mentor was different, though. He didn't punish him for his sensitivities, but let them flower and bloom; his eagerness was refreshing, and his interests and curiosity mirrored his own. He'd written glowing recommendations and helped send him on his six-year voyage. In those years he'd accomplished things his mentor hadn't... couldn't... left him wounded...

Can't you bend? he thought. Do you always have to be so perfect? Stand up to the system! Believe in yourself!

The ensuing days would offer the final hours of solidarity between them.

"Do you hear that?"

"Yes, I do."

"Mike, I know I've told you this a hundred times," Ethel said. "But when you read what you've written, the words just flow so...

"Was I the patient that you and Dr. Brand were examining?... I thought so. While you were reading I could see the three of us so clearly."

"There's another piece I just finished, Ethel. It's about my mentor in DC. Would you like to hear it?... I call it *Bennie - The Enigma.*"

Dr. Amin had unfathomable mechanical skill, and unrivaled anatomical expertise. I marveled at the intensity he brought to each and every patient. Observing him was like watching a symphony conductor fine-tune an orchestra. He had perfect pitch, and a feeling for every nuance of the body. At the hint of the slightest off-note, he'd go searching for the source of disharmony until the patient's system was perfectly in tune.

I quickly adapted to assisting him, and developed a feeling for when to ask questions, and when to be silent - When to offer my assistance, and when to step back.

The turning point came when Bennie brought me to examine a well-off Romanian man who complained of chest pain. He'd been to all the best specialists - None of whom could offer an explanation.

Bennie scanned him, then asked me to do the same.

A focus of energy radiated from his chest.

"Where in the chest? How deep is it?"

I don't know. How do I figure that out?

"Envision a ruler, then count through the inches. When you get to the right level, you'll feel the energy give out."

Why does it do that?

"Because you've temporarily reconciled the body with the source of injury by focusing your energy there...

"Pain is there to tell you something. It's the body's way of saying 'It's right here - Now do something about it'...

"When you address the wound, the body responds by saying, 'Oh, he's got the message' and turns down the volume."

I conceived a ruler - At three inches the energy faded.

"What kind of tissue is involved?... Lung or muscle?"

How do I determine that?

"Picture what muscle looks like and what lung is."

It was lung.

"Now, what is the process?"

What do you mean - "process"?

"Is it inflammation? Is it a scar? Is it a granuloma? Is it an infection? Visualize in your mind what each of these looks like."

It was a scar.

The patient said he'd been exposed to tuberculosis in his youth. He'd told his other doctors, but nothing had ever shown up on chest X-ray or CT, so they'd dismissed it.

Bennie explained that the scars from these infections are often so subtle they aren't seen on imaging studies. Nevertheless, they create significant tugs on the fascial planes, provoking misalignments and pain.

Bennie instructed the patient in the use of breathing exercises; on subsequent visits, he reported feeling better, his chest pain resolved.

This was my turning point. After being witness to and participant in these events my outlook on medicine would never be the same. I had discovered within myself the innate ability to diagnose and localize disease. This ability did not depend on laboratory or imaging findings; but simply attuning to the invisible signals of the body...

"Mike," she said, *"you just have so many talents. You just do. You have so many talents. All rolled up in one little package...*

"All the time that you were reading I just kept wondering what would happen next...

"Mike, would you ever publicize your work? I mean, who would you submit it to? Do you think others would benefit from it?"

"The thing I do - this bioenergy - is something that can help everyone - No matter what the injury.

"It works for everything. The whole world needs it. I could see hundreds of patients a day, and never tire."

"Yes," she said. "It's important to enjoy what you do."
But in her words I heard a note of doubt - And it left me feeling uncertain and insecure...

CHAPTER TWENTY-EIGHT

Sunday, October 5, 1997

I was going to the beach, and asked Ethel if she'd like to come along?

"Not today," she said. "I'm still having these stomach problems, and it seems like each one of the different medications I'm on is just making it worse."

"Yes, Ethel, I'm afraid that's true. The morphine causes nausea; Baritol increases acid and erodes the lining of the stomach; Lytec counters the effects of the Baritol, but causes cramping."

"Yes, I can feel all that," she said. "Especially with the Lytec."

I hesitated.

"Ethel, can I tell you something?... I worry about you so much."

Warm tears formed in my eyes and flowed down my cheeks.

"Oh, Mike, don't worry," she said. "I'm alright. It isn't that bad. I'm getting stronger. Oh, don't worry, Mike. Mike..."

The current was strong that evening, and a storm collected over the beach.

I was enjoying the ocean - Taken by the undertow to deeper waters - The waves crashing over my head.

When I looked back, the shoreline had disappeared, eclipsed by the rising tide.

Metal stairwells lined the cliffs, and I swam to the first one -

But the current pulled me past it, dragging me further out to sea.

The next stairwell came into view. I couldn't see another, and didn't know when I'd get another chance.

I navigated between the water and the rocks -
But, again, was pulled past.
I swam against the current, struggling to get back.
As I got closer the waves began to lift and throw me towards the cliff -
Clinging to the rocks, I lifted myself out of the water, and then scurried to the steps.
From the road I looked back - Admiring the purple skies, gray clouds and rugged sea...

"I brought this back from the beach for you, Ethel."
I held out a shell; most had been black, and saturated with oil; this one was white and thin and delicate.
"Ooh, that's nice, Mike."
She stood admiring it as though it were a precious gem, then crept to the entertainment center, and set it down next to the card I'd sent her.
"I got a sandwich from the health food store," I said. "I hope it's something you can eat."
"Oh, thank you, Mike. It smells delicious."
I went to the kitchen and looked through the cabinets for plates -
The only one left was covered in plastic.
"That's funny," I thought.
I unwrapped it -
It was the plate I'd given her in the hospital...

"When I was a little girl," she said, "I had long bushy eyebrows. And one day I got so tired of looking at them, Mike, that I just cut them - I mean I really cut them.

"When my aunt came home, and saw what I'd done, she punished me.

"She gave me a licking for it, and told me never to do it again... Oh, it wasn't anything like a whipping - I don't think I ever got one of those - Not like a lot of kids I knew. She just gave me a spanking and sent me to my room.

"The thing was, though, she only looked at one eye. She didn't see I'd cut the eyebrow over the other eye, too. And when she's sees it, she punishes me again.

"I was so mad. It's okay if I'm punished for something I did do. But punish me for something I didn't - Uh, uh.

"I got out a piece of paper and wrote it all down. Everything I was feeling.

"It was really funny. I was in my room, and my aunt was entertaining some guests; every time I came to a word I couldn't spell, I would call out to the others in the living room, 'How do you spell...?'

"When I finished, I ripped it up and threw it all away..."

"And do you know what, Mike?" she said, laughing. "Auntie took it out of the waste basket, and put the pieces back together - She gave me another licking then."

"I have a story, Ethel... Just after I'd gotten my driver's license I was driving home from a piano lesson, and a girl pulled out in front of me and hit my car.

"When I got home and told my mother, she didn't believe me -

"'Are you sure,' she says. 'It looks like you went into her.'"

"While we were in New York that summer, the girl's father sent us a letter - Saying they were taking us to court, and suing us for the damages. Still, no one in my family would believe my side of the story.

"It was tearing me up inside.

"One night I was sitting alone in the kitchen with the lights off - My grandfather came in, and asked me what was the matter?

"After I told him, he says, 'Michael, I want you to look at the table. Now imagine it represents the whole of human suffering.'

"'Your problem,' he said, 'doesn't even amount to a grain of salt.'"

"How did that make you feel?" Ethel said.

"Better. I didn't feel so bad anymore - Like my problem was so terrible, and I was the only one."

"How did the case turn out?"

"The judge ruled in my favor."

"What did your family say then?"

"They didn't say much - Takes a lot to impress my family..."

CHAPTER TWENTY-NINE

I went to Ethel's with a month's supply of medicines.
"Oh, thank you, Mike! You didn't have to do that..."
"I wanted to, Ethel. I'm worried about leaving..."
I broke off -
"I'd like to do some bioenergy before I go - But I wrote another short-story, and I wanted to share it with you."
"Okay, Mike."
"It's about my old girlfriend Elizabeth, who I'll be visiting during the trip. I call it *The Choice...*"

Elizabeth became my primary link to developing my skills as a healer. In particular, with Liz I could focus on those traumas I was most interested in - The emotional scars of childhood.

One day I'd been working to uncover the reason for her food allergies, using a technique Bennie taught me that involved following the fascial planes and assessing the body's response to questions.

The thought of anything to do with food, and her body immediately locked.

*I tried to get at the source, posing questions to the body -
Was it chemical? Emotional?*

Then, the thought of her father popped into my head, and, immediately, the tension in her body released. I asked if she felt something different; she said she was experiencing an uncomfortable lump in her throat.

Focusing on her father, I probed deeper. Soon, the glide in her fascial planes was normal, and free of any tension on the matter of food allergies. Her throat cleared, as she remained completely loose.

I told Elizabeth what happened, and she recounted how parsimonious her father had been with food. He'd lived through the depression, and nearly went hungry. In turn, he had all but starved his children - Perhaps because he wanted his children to suffer the way he did. Maybe it was no coincidence that she and her three sisters suffered from some form of gastro-intestinal illness, she said...

That night Elizabeth had a migraine, and wanted me to stay up and comfort her - And I just didn't want to do that! I could handle doing something productive like bioenergy or cranial sacral therapy. But staying up all night doing nothing?! - The whole thing left me tired; I lay down and went to sleep.

Elizabeth was angry. She told me she didn't need all my high-powered therapies and psychological theories. What she needed was a little TLC - Attention - Emotional support. She said maybe the reason so many of Dr. Amin's patients got worse when they left the clinic [Something I'd been ruminating over for months] was because their homes weren't warm, nurturing places, and didn't give them that degree of added support they needed to get better.

Maybe it didn't take primal therapy on everyone who walked through Dr. Amin's doors to enable them to recover from their childhood wounds, she said. Perhaps, it was a whole lot simpler than I ever imagined. Maybe all they really needed was a little tenderness and affection in their lives.

That's what she thought she needed, she said. Instead of me reasoning with her why she should feel alright, maybe I could just hold her and pamper her - Just a little - Once in a while.

It wasn't peoples' fault they didn't have good Mommies and Daddies, she said. And maybe it isn't so bad they go looking for a Mommy and Daddy later in life to supply those needs that weren't met in childhood.

Couldn't I just hold her, and love her even when she was feeling low - Just support her in those times she needed me...

"It just flows so," Ethel said. "I know I've told you this so many times - But when you read what you've written it just flows so nicely. I just want it to go on and on..."

I held out my hand.

Ethel smiled, and closed her eyes - Her fingertips caressing my palm.

"It's interesting, Ethel. I'm feeling a lot of sensations on the left side of my head..."

"Is that okay, Mike?"

"Oh, yes, Ethel. It feels like it's trying to get at an old wound...

"It's funny. I've always had problems on that side. I think it started when I was a boy -

"I'd been playing outside when one of the neighbor kids threw a toy truck at me...

"I ran and jumped on top of him, and hit him on the head the way he'd hit me.

"He cried, and begged me to stop -

"But I wouldn't - I couldn't - I just had to hurt him as much as he hurt me..."

Just then, the muscles in my head twitched, and the entire side released.

"Ethel, some kind of healing's taking place - *Without me even trying - And I don't know why.*"

I opened my eyes.

She sat smiling, eyes full of care and warmth.

"Ethel, can I tell you something?... This trip to the east coast - Well, there are people I can visit - Places I can see - *But, really, my heart is here.*"

She dipped her head, and suppressed her smile.

"I think it will be good for you, Mike," she said, regaining her composure. *"You can get yourself refreshed...*

"You could see that friend of yours. What's her name?... Elizabeth - I'm sure it would cheer her up - Seeing you..."

CHAPTER THIRTY

Al was waiting when I arrived in DC.

We went to Great Falls, and sat on the rocks overlooking the water.

"It was like I could feel what they were feeling," I said. "Or at least pinpoint in their bodies where the lesions were."

"In that case," he said, "it sounds like you transferred the person's energy field to your own body."

Of course, I thought. Interlink.

"When you reach a state at which the frequency of motion exactly corresponds to the oscillations you're providing, the molecules vibrate at their maximal capacity," he continued. "That's the resonant frequency..."

For years I'd been searching to take bioenergy to a higher level - One that wouldn't rely on scanning, but communicate the needs of the person directly.

It had been there all along, I thought. Why hadn't it occurred to me earlier?...

We drove to the fisherman's wharf, and bought a half-barrel of blue crab.

After dinner we sat on his patio overlooking Potomac.

"Bioenergy seems to be helping Ethel with her discomfort," I said. "But I wonder if it isn't working on her cancer, as well."

"Mike, do you really believe bioenergy can work for something like cancer? It sounds a little far-fetched to me."

"The way I see it, Al, cancer represents nothing more than a breakdown in communication between the body and its cells.

"I mean, what are we? This conglomeration of cells - Come together to work for the common good.

"It took hundreds of millions of years to evolve to this state from a single-celled organism.

"To do this, the cells had to form a pact - One that said they'd be willing to sacrifice themselves for the good of the whole.

"In most forms of cancer, though, you find is a collection of cells that have run amok, and keep growing despite the harm they cause to the body.

"The question is 'Why?' - Why don't cancer cells abide by the 'All for one' principle? How is it that they bring about the destruction of the very organism that their survival depends?

"The answer seems to be that they're *reacting* to something.

"Most cancers develop in response to toxins. The person is smoking or drinking, and generating free radicals that result in mutations in the DNA.

"In the case of most cells, suicide pathways are activated, so the cell can self-destruct rather than transform into something malignant.

"But what if the cells of your body get tired of the same abuses - Say, 'Hey, why should I lay my life down for you? You're just trying to kill yourself. I'm gonna do my own thing?'

"So, with time and more toxic exposures, mutations develop and enable these cells to tap into their single-cell memory - One that will permit them to live as their ancestors did - Independent - Not relying on other cells.

"We evolved from single-celled organisms - Why shouldn't the blue-prints for that machinery still be there -

"Chemotherapy can kill most of these cells initially - But, usually, some cancer cells survive. And is it any wonder? It's just the same message - 'I'm exposing you to toxins - I'm trying to kill you.'

"That's where bioenergy comes in. Perhaps, through bioenergy, a communication can be effected - Say to the cancer cell, 'The person's sorry for what he or she's done in the past, and isn't going to do it again -

"'Now it's your turn - Activate what's left of your self-destruct mechanisms so the body can heal.'

"In this way the tumor can regress, and the person's health be restored."

The sun had set -

Al sat silent in the shadows.

"You know, when you say it like that, Mike," he said. "I agree with you..."

CHAPTER THIRTY-ONE

I took the Metro to Alexandria, and met Don at his office on King Street.

"Hey there."

He greeted me with an expansive handshake and hug.

We talked on our way to a crowded Thai restaurant, and were seated in a booth in the back.

"So what about this woman you wrote me about... Ethel?" he said. "Do you like her more than Liz?"

"I don't think it's a matter of liking her more - They're different. Liz loved me for my potential - What I could be. Ethel likes me for who I am - Now - In the present..."

"That's what's important, though! The present!"

"I don't agree. Elizabeth worked to make me better, and see things in a different way. Everything I've done - Who I am, what I've become - is a direct result of her."

"Don't misunderstand me," he said. "I know Liz had an important effect on your life. But where you are now, you're going to make those changes no matter what you do. It's a part of your destiny...

"Over the past months I have been studying Buddhism, and trying to learn the importance of letting life's events unfold by themselves - You know how difficult that is for me! Look at what I do for a living! I'm an architect. A planner! I plan everything to the minutest detail. It has taken me a long time to learn to step back and look at things from a distance. But I've found my life is a whole lot more content when I do."

"Don, the way I see it, within our lives we live in different realities. A huge part of my reality is the feeling that, at its core, this life represents nothing more than a spiritual entity experiencing the lessons of the universe on a physical plane - Like the difference between learning something firsthand and reading it in a book.

"But, then, there's another reality as well - One that's lived in the moment - When you stand in the thick of things, and really get involved..."

"This woman Ethel - I don't know..." I said, breaking-off. "I cherish her so much. I just want our relationship to go on and on..."

"And are you willing, then, to let this person go?" he said.

A detached feeling crept over me.

"No," I said. "No. I don't want her to die."

"Then it's your problem," he said...

CHAPTER THIRTY-TWO

Saturday, October 18, 1997

Elizabeth was waiting when I got off the plane in Providence...

"I'm always struck by the how un-intimate it is when we make love," she said. *"It's very physical - and you know I love that - But there's no emotion in it. You don't say things. I don't know how you feel - even after all this time. How do you feel about me?"*

"You're a person who loves me," I said, "and pushes me to reach my potential."

A look of disappointment swept her features.

"I know that - And there's nothing really wrong with our relationship. But I want something different now. I want affection. I want love. Why is it so difficult for you to give me that?..."

The next day we went to her mother's -

Her sister Tanya was there, with her husband Brandon and two year old daughter Calie.

The toddler roamed the house - Looking at the world with thought-filled eyes, and not at all sure what she saw.

When she flashed a worried look at me, I stared back -

"What do you want?" I thought. *"What can I do?"*

Brandon and Tanya came and embraced Calie, and met her unsure expression with smiles and laughter.

Elizabeth crept behind me -

"Think of the things you would have done," she said, *"had the people around you when you were growing up said 'Yes' to you, and smiled at everything you did."*

I hesitated.

"I don't know, Liz," I said. "I mean, I have my PhD - I'm on my way to getting my MD. What else would I have been?"

"Happy!" she said in her perky style. "For one thing..."

CHAPTER THIRTY-THREE

I called Ethel when I got off the plane in Streeport.

"I have an appointment at the Neurology clinic tomorrow at nine," she said. "I wonder if they can tell me something about the problems I've been having, and if it has something to do with my MS?..."

The next morning I sat in the clinic waiting for her -

But at ten o'clock she still wasn't there...

"My daughter and I had gotten our signals crossed," she said. "She thought I needed a ride in the afternoon instead of the morning, and now she's busy...

"I guess I'll have to call a taxi."

"I'll pick you up, Ethel," I said. "Just give me a few minutes..."

I pulled up at her apartment -

The door was open, and Ethel was inside nervously puffing on a cigarette.

She put on her black leather coat, and met me at the car.

"How are you, Ethel?"

"Fine, Mike."

She stared ahead -

I thought she looked uncomfortable.

"The change in seasons in New England was really beautiful," I said. "We drove by grooves of maple trees, all of them different colors - Leaves yellow and red and orange."

Ethel continued looking out in front of her -

I didn't think she was listening...

The wind blew through the barren medical center.

"Ethel, I'm going to let you out in front of the entrance. I'll park the car and meet you inside."

When I arrived at the clinic, Ethel was perched on a chair in the corner, looking about like a child in an unfamiliar place.

How is it that she could look so vulnerable? I thought...

Ethel was drawn up in a corner as the Neurologists stood over her.

"I'm at a loss to explain her symptoms," said one. "I suppose there are some medications we could give her if we think it's related to her MS..."

After the appointment Ethel had to go to the pharmacy to get some medications.

I was sure it would be a two-hour wait.

"Mike, Shoniah can pick me up if you have things you need to do."

"Are you sure, Ethel?"

"Yes, Mike."

She opened her purse and dug for a few dollars.

"Here, Mike. This is for the parking."

"No, that's okay, Ethel..."

"Please! Please!" she insisted...

That evening I stared up from my books, feeling sad I'd left her...

"Oh, hi, Mike," she said. "I was thinking about you on the ride home from the hospital...

"Shon picked me up, and on the way I was noticing all the different colors of the leaves on the plants and trees, and thinking, 'We have a change of seasons here, too..."

CHAPTER THIRTY-FOUR

On Saturday morning the streets were quiet, and when the door opened at Ethel's, the room felt full of light.

"Mike, I have several members of my family over," Ethel said. "Let me introduce you...

"I'd like you to meet my mother, Mrs. Small."

Rosy-cheeked, and eyes that looked like they were bubbling over, she didn't speak.

"This is my sister Janet."

She sat lounging on the couch.

"Everything is so polluted now," she said, in between puffs on a cigarette. "And nothing is good for you anymore..."

"This is my Aunt Belle."

A meek woman, she smiled and spoke quietly.

Ethel had told me Auntie didn't seem to age -

There was a photo of her on the mantelpiece; Shoniah was in the picture, and couldn't have been more than six ; Auntie looked even older then...

"And this is my father, Mr. Isaiah."

Isaiah Small was her stepfather. He'd been a contractor, and built many of the large estates in Streeport's Riverwalk district.

Short in stature, he appeared a man of immense strength, with compact build, powerful protruding abdomen, and well-arched back.

His legs were bowed, and steps utterly silent.

Redundant folds of skin met between his brows and protruded from his forehead.

His nose was Romanesque and distinguished-looking, though his expression humble.

Most striking were his hands -

Powerful and large, they looked like they belonged to a giant...

"Oh, and this is Uncle Jack."

Thin as a rail and proper, he took short swift steps in my direction.

"I hear you're a great friend of Ethel's," he said, "and the two of you worked together."

It took me a moment to realize he meant the CPR classes -

"Uh, uh, uh," I said.

"'Uh, uh, uh', he says," looking over his shoulder at the others...

Mr. Small took Uncle Jack home -

Ethel left with Janet, Auntie Belle and her cousin Gina for the store.

Ethel smiled and waved as she and the others drove past.

I stood alongside her mother and waved back.

"She asked me if I would come over, and stay with her for a few days," Mrs. Small said. "I'd rather that she come to my place in the country, but she doesn't want to.

"She's been doing a lot better since I come over. I think I do as much for her as the medicines."

"There are different kinds of medicines, Mrs. Small," I said. "They don't all come in a bottle."

She stood placid and stony-silent -

I didn't think she understood, and decided there wasn't much there.

"She needs love right now!" she said firmly. "That's why I'm so happy you're here!..."

CHAPTER THIRTY-FIVE

In the evening Ethel and I sat in the dim light of her kitchen.

"My first husband and I had known each other from the time we were children in school," she said. "We married young. I tried to do the things I thought he'd like, and would make a man happy. But he was always off somewhere sowing his oats...

"We married too young...

"My second husband, Ivy's dad, was immature. He had to have everything his way. He still calls his mother when he wants something. She goes and gets it for him!...

"In between marriages, there was always Matthew...

"But our approaches to things like child raising were too different, and we couldn't get along...

"He doesn't deal well with illness - I'm surprised he hasn't actually stayed away more than he has. His brother died of a bleeding ulcer. Matthew himself has problems. Once he had to be hospitalized when an ulcer bled."

"Ethel, just because Matthew's had some bad experiences doesn't excuse him from not being there for others.

"He's got to grow up and learn how to care."

A confused titillating smile played upon her features - As though she were on the verge of some understanding, but not quite there yet.

"What did you say, Mike?"

"I said, 'He has to learn how to care.'"

The bewildered expression persisted, and she turned her head...

CHAPTER THIRTY-SIX

Ethel's blood count was falling, and she was scheduled to have a transfusion.

In a dream I saw her suspended naked by IV lines connected to flasks of blood, with only a sheet the size of a face cloth to cover her -

Again and again she struggled to disentangle her arm from the lines, and pulled at the cloth to better conceal herself.

"Ethel, don't worry about that," I thought. "It's not so important."

But she wouldn't stop -

As though preserving her modesty were as important as her predicament...

CHAPTER THIRTY-SEVEN

Friday, November 7, 1997

A follow up CT scan had been performed to assess Ethel's response to chemotherapy.

I went to the file room, and asked for her films -

The cancer was growing -

Small tumors in her liver, barely perceptible two months earlier, were larger, and there were many more of them -

In the center of her abdomen was an indefinable mass - crowding and swallowing the other organs...

"Ethel, can I read you something... It's some free-verse I wrote about my upper level John Wang?"

"Yes, Mike. Was he the resident I met that day I saw you coming out of the Claude Ray?"

"That's right, Ethel. I call it, *Who would move mountains.*

On a Sunday morning
The short white-jacketed figure
Emerged from the Hospital
With his favorite resident.
A combination of Asian upbringing,
And Western thought,
Melded into a presence of mind,
And unyielding force of will.
He could move mountains,
Would he?
'I need you to help me grow.'

'I can't be everything for you.'
Tension and resentment mounted
Pulled them apart
But walking into the morning sun
Their tour of duty behind them
Neither could deny
He liked the other.
'How will you get on?!
'I see so much in you!
'Will you rise to the challenge that confronts you?!'

"Mike, when you read what you've written, *the words just flow so...*"

She was so full of life.
I stared into the lightbox.
Have I been in denial?
A feeling of self-containment enveloped me -
Like being enclosed in a bubble -
With no way of breaking through...

CHAPTER THIRTY-EIGHT

Sunday, November 16, 1997

Ethel and I sat doing bioenergy at her kitchen table.

Energy beamed from the top of my head - Bristling from my scalp.

I closed my eyes, and immersed myself in the feeling.

"Mike, are you alright?" Ethel said.

"Yes, I'm alright, Ethel." My eyes still shut. "Why do you ask?"

"I don't know - It's just that you look really *sad.*"

"Oh, I'm sorry, Ethel. I guess I should have said something, but I figured the stuff I do is strange enough without me saying 'It feels like I'm being gripped by energy and it's actively working on something inside of me.'"

"I was just concerned - Because you looked so *sad.*"

"It's a good thing, Ethel. I feel like it's getting at an old wound."

"It's not the first time I've seen you look this way," she said. "From the first time we did this together, I saw that look come over you... *And every time since.*"

I gazed downwards.

"I wonder, Ethel - Maybe at the core of my being I'm a sad person."

She hesitated, and I could feel her pull back...

That evening I phoned Elizabeth -

"You used to do that same thing with me, too!" she said. "We'd be sitting there talking at the kitchen table, and, all of a sudden, your face would go blank with no explanation!...

"You can't do that to people! You can't assume they know what you're feeling! You have to tell them!...

"But I don't think it's a matter of being a sad person - I think it has more to do with you being blocked..."

The next morning I awoke to a feeling of being fully charged -
My heart radiated outward, expanding in my chest -
My head beamed with energy -
I felt ready for anything - Impatient for challenges that lay ahead.
I reached for the phone...
"Oh, hi, Mike," she said.
Her tone was distracted.
"I'm fine."
She sounded far away.
I tried to make conversation -
Her voice didn't change.
"I'll let you go, Ethel," I said.
"Okay, Mike."
I put down the receiver -
Unlike all the other times, she didn't ask me to call back.

CHAPTER THIRTY-NINE

On Thanksgiving I sat studying at my desk.

Organizing my papers I came across a stray entry from my diary.

I didn't call Ethel tonight. I let my insecurities ('Am I calling her too often?') get the better of me. Now I feel terrible. It's just like me to pull back from a really good thing. And - on today - her first day of chemotherapy!...

I'd talked to her the night before -

"I called Dr. Brand last night," she'd said. "He had given me his phone number, and told me to call him if I had any questions...

"I told him about the sleeping problems I've been having, and he asked me what medicines I had. I told him I had some valium that I'd been prescribed for my MS, and he said maybe I could I take one before going to bed. It worked. It was the first time in a while that I got a full night's rest..."

"That's great, Ethel," I'd said -

But, really, I felt outdone...

Elizabeth phoned -

"Are you going to have dinner with anyone today, Mike?"

"Ethel had invited me over, but I don't think I'll go?"

"Why not, Mike?"

"She's kind of distant - I don't feel appreciated anymore..."

"Mike, try to put your feet in her shoes, and see how you'd cope with it!...

"She's dying, Mike! Dying! Do you know what that is?! Do you know what that must feel like?!...

"In many ways she's dying for your benefit! - Because she's permitting you into her life! - She's giving you a chance to experience something in a way you'll probably never experience it again, and yet will be called upon to oversee people dying many, many times in your career!...

"You owe it to her to be good to her - Because really the person who benefits most from this experience is you!...

"She's dying, Mike! She doesn't get a second chance!

"But you do! - And she's the one giving it to you!..."

I arrived at Ethel's midday.

Shoniah met me at the door.

"Mom's upstairs getting dressed," she said. "Let me introduce you to some of the family you haven't met yet..."

Mrs. Small came over.

"How you doin', Mikie?! Get yourself a plate, and have something!"

I sat on the floor, and played with Sammy - Mindful that he didn't bump his head on the glass coffee table behind him...

"Mike... Mike..."

A voice resonated inside me -

"Mike... Mike..."

It flowed over me -

"Mike... Mike..."

Bathing me in its soothing quality -

"Mike?..."

I turned.

There was Ethel - Wearing a modest blue blouse - Smiling and vibrant.

"He didn't even know you were there!" Uncle Jack called out, laughing.

She dipped her head, and held back her laughter.

I just looked up, and smiled...

CHAPTER FORTY

I deliberately let a few days pass before calling Ethel again.

She'd looked so well during the Thanksgiving dinner; I didn't want to burden her with my concern.

I called on Saturday morning.

"I'm experiencing worsening pain," she said. *"I haven't slept or eaten in the past two days, and, now, there's this new pain that's developed..."*

Her voice was anxious, on the verge of tears.

"I don't know, Mike. I don't know what to do."

"Would you like me to come over, Ethel, and see what I can do?"

"If you want to..."

She gasped and broke off, sobbing...

Her mother met me at the door -

Without a word, she escorted me upstairs.

Ethel was slumped over in bed.

"Hi, Mike," she said, lifting her head.

"Hi, Ethel."

Janet stepped out of the shadows, smiling as though pleased with herself.

"Mike, I have a question," she said. "Whose decision is it to take her to the hospital?"

"It's hers," I said.

"She says she doesn't want to go, and I think she has to..."

"I don't want to go to the hospital, Janet," Ethel interrupted, *straining to speak in a pleasant tone. "I'm not comfortable there. I'd rather be in my own home."*

"You see! She doesn't want to go!..."

Janet promptly left; Ethel followed her with her eyes; hurt and disappointed; frail and weak.

"Where is it hurting, Ethel?"

"All down my back. In my stomach. My chest."

"Let's see what we can do."

Positioning myself behind her I laid my hands on her back -

Through the nightgown I could feel the tight muscles -

Then, with the slightest pressure, the knots melted away...

One by one I followed them.

I looked at the clock on the dresser -

The minutes passed -

Then the hours -

As the light in the room began to fade.

I leaned forward -

Resting my head on her back -

Breathing the scent of her freshly washed robe -

Moving with her rhythmic breathing -

Her body so emaciated, I could feel every rib...

"Thank you, Mike. I'm feeling much better."

"Do you feel like eating something, Ethel?"

"I'd like to have some ribs. Shoniah brought some over from Luther's yesterday."

"I'll get them."

I went to the refrigerator, and put the ribs on a plate...

"Mike, I can't eat these," she said. "They're all cold."

"Oh, sorry, Ethel - Whenever I have leftover ribs, I like them straight out of the refrigerator."

She smiled, and shook her head.

"I'll be right back..."

Ethel rested.

I went downstairs and picked up a book of children's Bible stories - The same as I'd been given.

I looked at the inscription on the jacket -

"To Ivy From Mommie".

I felt a pair of eyes, peering at me through the dark -

I looked up and saw Aunt Belle - So silent in the sparsely lit room I hadn't noticed her before.

She smiled at my startled expression, and lunged forward and kissed me...

I went back upstairs.

"How are you feeling, Ethel?"
"I feel better, Mike. Thanks."
"I'm glad..."
I bent low, and kissed her.
Her hands fluttered like the wings of a butterfly on my back.
Leaving I caught sight of her reflection in the mirror -
Eyes closed and directed downwards -
Features soft and lit amidst her smile -
More beautiful than I'd ever seen her...

The rainy drive home I could still feel her skin on my lips -
Like I was a school-boy, just planted his first kiss...

The next day I left a note for Dr. Brand -

I spent Thanksgiving with Ethel. She talked about how much she appreciated your advice.

She spoke with deep affection and concern for your three-year old son recently diagnosed with diabetes.

She is a truly remarkable woman, Dr. Brand. I wish you could know her better ...

CHAPTER FORTY-ONE

The following weekend I'd been over at Ethel's when Shoniah came with Sammy.

Ethel sat up in bed -

"Sammy... Come to Grandma... Sammy..."

But the toddler scurried about, oblivious to her outstretched arms.

"Oh, well. Maybe you'll spend some time with Grandma later..."

Ivy came home from work.

"Hi, Sammy!" She scooped him up. "Has the baby been fed yet?... I want to feed him..."

She sat him on her lap, and spoon-fed him.

"That's the way you guys need to be taking care of your mother," I said.

Ethel lowered her head and suppressed a smile.

"You mean just like that?!" Ivy whipped back.

"Whatever it takes," I said...

That evening the family gathered to watch a video.

Shoniah stood behind her mother, embroidering her hair with long threads.

"What are you doing?" I asked.

"Braiding Mom's hair," Shoniah responded.

"I've been losing a lot of hair because of the chemotherapy I'm getting," Ethel said. "Shoniah and I talked about what we could do, and decided that braiding my hair would make it look nicer..."

The movie was about a woman's pursuit of a man I found shallow.

"Oh, I can't stand this guy!" I called out.

"Why not, Mike?" Ethel said.
"He's so full of himself!" I snapped back.
Ethel suppressed a smile, and lowered her head...

"When I accepted Christ," Shoniah said, "I knew I was saved."
"Saved from what?" I said.
"Saved," she said. "Just saved."
"Mike, what do you believe in?" Ethel asked.
"I have my own religion, Ethel."
"But you're Christian, right?"
"No, Ethel. I'm Jewish."
"What's 'Jewish'," she said, with an amused half-smile. "What do Jewish people believe in?"
I shrugged my shoulders -
"One God - 'Do unto others as you would have them do unto you.' - Jesus was Jewish...
"Anyway, I have my own thoughts on spirituality... A combination of chaos theory and the idea that everything is important and impacts on everything else, and Buddhism and the aspiration towards nothingness...
"I believe when I lose myself in others, I get more connected to the whole."
The room fell silent.
"I suppose my conversion happened one evening when I saw my friend Elizabeth burst into light."
"What happened?" Shoniah said.
"We were at my friend Al's house. The three of us would get together on the weekends, and practice Chi Gong in his basement.
"Elizabeth and Al had been talking for a long time. I was tired, so when the two of them got up to practice, and told them to go on without me.
"Then, just as they were about to start, Elizabeth turns around, and says, 'Mike, watch my aura.'
"I had had a couple of experiences seeing auras.
"I said, 'Okay,' and sat back on the couch.
"They begin to practice, and - sure enough - I see Liz's aura. It looks like this thick film of buzzy gray stuff coming off all around her.
"She's patting herself - Her head, her shoulders, her chest - And this gray film seems to be moving down into the ground.
"I'm thinking, 'Good, she's getting rid of a lot of bad energy - Turbid chi - I bet she's going to feel a lot better after this.'

"Then - Out of nowhere - There's this burst of white light that comes flashing out of her! Just for a second - Bang! - Like a firefly, or quick explosion!

"And it's white! - A flash of white light!...

"I jumped back in the couch - I'm thinking, 'Whoa! What was that?!'

"Meanwhile, Elizabeth's trembling all over. She motions me over with her hands - She's so terrified she can hardly speak.

"She tells me to hold her - Al, too. She says she feels cold, and seen something that's really scared her.

"Then she tells us her vision -

"She said she saw herself carrying her dead body from a past life to a lot of fluffy, happy-go-lucky creatures that take the body, and tell her to be on her way.

"She's filled with questions, though -

"'What happened?' she asks them. 'What does this mean?'

"But the creatures pay her no mind - 'Shoo - Scoot,' they say. 'It's nothing - Go back to your life...'"

"Well, that's it, I guess. I really don't understand it - I only know I can't deny what I saw."

Shoniah stood staring.

Ethel's eyes were closed; head lowered; a suppressed smile on her lips...

CHAPTER FORTY-TWO

Sunday, December 21, 1997

I was leaving for the east coast to spend the holiday with Elizabeth and her family.

Ethel was very sick now, and hadn't slept in two days.

I put my hand on her abdomen -

It felt stiff - Like leather pulled over a drum.

I scanned her -

Just above the navel, a bubble of energy enveloped my hand and lead me through a downward spiral, till dissipating into the ground.

I felt her abdomen again - It was less stiff.

I guided my hand in clockwise circles.

Her hand held her gown, and with each cycle her fingertips caressed my hand.

I peered into her face.

Her features were hard now - Like the figures from Van Gogh's *Potato Eaters*.

She drifted off - Her head bobbing, as she tried to stay awake.

The night before she'd bruised her forehead when she bumped into a door.

I eyed the bruise, then scanned it energetically.

The energy drew me closer, until I lightly caressed her.

She awoke with a start, and pulled her legs to her chest.

I thought she felt uncomfortable, and collected my things...

"I never thought it would happen this way," she said. "I never thought it would happen - That I would be alone and sick - Other

people, maybe - But not to me - I didn't think it would happen to me - Not that way - Not me."

Her voice was warm and enchanting -
I could envision her smiling.
"And now it's happened..."

Michael Yanuck MD PhD

PART TWO

Michael Yanuck MD PhD

CHAPTER FORTY-THREE

During the holiday I visited craft shops, looking for gifts for Elizabeth and her family.

In one shop I found a pair of ear-rings -

Shaped like dangling triangles, they were entirely composed of tiny beads, black and white and orange -

"What a lovely gift they'd be for Ethel," I thought.

But I'd already given her a present before leaving Streeport.

I didn't need to get her two...

I left the shop.

For the rest of the day, the ear-rings called to me...

"They're beautiful, Mike!"

She let the ear-rings dangle, eyes aglow.

"They're just like something I would have bought for myself..."

"They had you're name written all over them, Ethel. They wouldn't let me leave without them..."

"Oh, thank you, Mike!"

She flew over and kissed me -

Her lips and touch were so gentle they felt like a wisp of air on my cheek...

"Mike, I have some meat that I just thawed. I know you came here to work on my back, but would you mind if I cooked dinner first..."

We sat and watched a made-for-television movie, like the ones I used to watch on nights my mother would go out, and I'd be at home with babysitters.

I hadn't seen one in years, and it struck me how much I'd enjoyed them -

Now, I sat probing the screen, dissecting every line and nuance.

I gazed over at Ethel -

Eyes unassuming -

Wholly without criticism or harsh thought.

"What is keeping me from enjoying this?..."

Sunlight filled the living room -

"He was beautiful, Mike," she said. *"He was a Doberman pincher - The only dog I ever owned...*

"And, do you know, Mike, when he would come and sit on the couch, he would sit the way we do... With his rear-end on the seat, and his legs hanging over..."

I burst out laughing.

"I'm sorry, Ethel - I just got the image of a dog with a beer can watching the game."

"Yeah, just like that. He'd just sit there on the couch like everyone else...

"This dog was so smart, Mike. He never hurt the children, even when they would annoy him...

"This was especially true of Kim. She'd be wanting to play with him and that sort of thing; he'd just come in and look at me - like he were saying, 'Would you please get this child away from me'..."

"I was on my way home," she said, "when I feel this guy running to me... I just saw him out of the corner of my eye. He was across the street a block away. But have you ever had the feeling that someone's after you? - Like they're looking at you, and want to get a hold of you? - That's what this felt like.

"I'd actually seen him the day before. I lived in a second story apartment at the time, and I could actually see him from over the fence, and feel him watching me.

"Well, I got out of my car, and he was standing there in front of me.

"He took hold of my wrists, and said, *'Come with me.'*

"I decided I would stay calm. There was no one else around, and I didn't want to make things any worse by yelling, because I didn't know what he'd do then.

"My apartment was just upstairs, and I thought if I could just get him to go up there, maybe I could make a break at the door, and call the police.

"So I said, *'Okay, but what if we go to my place?'*

"Just, then, one of my neighbors pulls up in his car.

"When he looks over, I broke away, and flew up the stairs to my apartment."

She began laughing -

"And do you know what, Mike?... He keeps standing down there... And he calls up to me, 'Is it still alright for me to come in?'"

She smiled broadly.

"I stood in my doorway, and called him every name in the book!..."

I'd been in my mother's room -

She'd been quizzing me for a spelling test when a man called.

She got off the phone.

"What do you think?" she said. "Should I go out with this guy? I told him I was helping you study for your test."

"I'm okay, mom," I said. "Have a good time."

The next morning she was upset.

"What's the matter, mom?"

"That guy you told me to go out with last night took me back to his apartment and showed me his dick.

"He had all kinds of locks on the door, and I was afraid I wouldn't get out.

"He takes out his dick in front of me, and says, 'Isn't this a great dick. Don't you think this is a great dick?' He said he did layouts for Playgirl magazine...

"I told him, 'I think I'd like to go home now.'

"On the way home, he drove real fast.

"I said, 'You're driving kinda fast.'

"'Who cares,' he says."

"I'm sorry, mom."

"And it's all your fault! - Because if you hadn't told me to go out with him, none of this would have happened!..."

Ethel sat shaking her head, smiling.

"I guess it was lucky that neighbor pulled up," she said. "If he hadn't, there might have been - Well - A problem."

"Ethel," I said. "You do have a way with understatement..."

"I used to think the most important thing in life was work," I said.

"I love my patients - They give me so much.

"But I wonder now... I wonder if finding my own happiness isn't important."

"I don't think there's anything more important than happiness," she responded spiritedly. *"I always thought, 'What I want most out of life is to be happy.'*

"I don't need to own a lot of fancy, expensive things and conveniences. I don't want that.

"I know people think I'm silly when I tell them - But I'd rather live up in a tree house with someone - And just be happy together!..."

CHAPTER FORTY-FOUR

Streeport was in the throes of its worst storm of the season.

I sat at my desk enjoying a view of the lightning - Striking the city and lighting up the skyline.

The phone rang.

"I'm experiencing worsening pain," Ethel said, *"and I just don't know what to do."*

"Have you taken your medications, Ethel?"

"Yes, but they don't seem to be having any effect."

"Do you want me to come out there, Ethel, and work on your back?"

"I don't know, Mike," she said tearfully. *"I know the weather's bad."*

I hesitated.

"Do you think it will help?"

"It's always helped before."

I looked outside.

"I don't know if I can get out there, Ethel. The streets are flooded. Can it wait till tomorrow?"

"Yes, Mike... That's okay... I'll be alright... Bye."

I stared at the pouring rain.

Shit, Mike. She wouldn't have called if it weren't serious!

You treated her just like Dr. Hood!... Like she was your patient!... Like you were her doctor!

I pulled on a raincoat, and bolted through the door...

Most of the streets were flooded, and the main road was closed; the detour led me through one narrow side street after another.

At Ethel's apartment the phone at the gate was dead.

115

A security officer stepped out of the guard booth -
He stood like a mountain - The torrential rains spilling over the brim of his hat like a waterfall.
He watched as I re-dialed Ethel's number.
"Will you please help me?"
Suddenly, he leapt into action - Buzzing open the gate before diving back into the guardhouse for shelter...

The short walk from the car to the apartment left me drenched.
"Look, it's Mike!" Ivy shouted. "Momma, Mike came!"
Dressed in a black Satin gown, hands dug into her sides, Ethel paced back and forth.
"If I could just get some relief - Some relief," she stammered. *"If I could just get some relief."*
I waited.
A demure smile graced her lips, as she passed -
Something I'd seen before -
In the throes of pain or tragedy - Some are able to let down their defenses - Effecting the most beautiful transformations - As they assume the identity of their true selves...

I suggested she take more medicine.
"I don't like to take more than the prescribed amount," she argued meekly.
"It will be alright, Ethel. You need it..."

With time she was able to sit and let me work on her -
But her muscles didn't relax like before...
In the end she slumped forward, and fell into an exhausted sleep...
I got up from the bed, and looked back -
Draped over a large cushioned pillow, she reminded me of *The Flaming June...*
I knelt beside her, and put my hand on her back -
She didn't stir.
I thought about the times I'd wanted to be with her -
But what if she awoke and felt uncomfortable? What if this should happen again, and she wasn't able to ask for my help?...

Standing at the top of the stairs I felt I hadn't done enough -
But I have to conserve my strength! I thought. The same thing can happen tomorrow! Who knows how long this will go on?!...
I lingered downstairs, and considered sleeping on the couch.

Perhaps she'll need me in the middle of the night?
But, again, I was afraid she'd feel uncomfortable -
"Besides," I told myself, "There are things to do in the morning - Appointments to keep..."

No harm come, I thought, as I closed the locked door behind me.
There was only a drizzle in the air now -
But driving home I hit a stretch of high water that tore out the underside of my car, and jammed it into the front tire...
As the sun rose I lay in a puddle -
My hands beet red and bleeding...

"I awoke after you'd gone," she said. "I called 'Mike... Mike...'
"Then I looked out through the window -
"Just in time to watch your white car pull away..."

CHAPTER FORTY-FIVE

Ethel checked into the hospital the next day.

She was admitted to Dr. Hines' service - The same team that had originally diagnosed her cancer.

"When Dr. Hines came by on rounds this morning," Ethel said, *"he didn't recognize me, or remember who I was...*

"I was surprised, because you think you'd remember someone who you told they had cancer to..."

The Oncology service had been consulted.

I rushed to attend rounds with Dr. Hood...

"I discussed this case with the fellow," a medical student said, "and we think that only supportive care measures are warranted, and adjustment of her pain control..."

Dr. Hood turned to me.

"Is there anything else you'd like to add, Mike?"

"Ethel's losing weight and having trouble getting food down. What do you think about the possibility of G-tube placement?..."

The oncology fellow interrupted.

"She is losing weight because of malignancy," he said.

He had handsome features, dark skin and moon blue-gray eyes.

"She has hypoalbuminemia," I said.

"Tumor necrosis factors can account for the laboratory findings," he flipped back.

"But it could be because she's malnourished."

"Unlikely," he said under his breath.

"She's not eating!" I said.

"G-tube has no reported prognostic significance in pancreatic cancer."

He'd responded without a moment's hesitation.

I looked at him stunned.

"'No prognostic significance,'" I thought. "This is a human being were talking about."

Dr. Hood broke the silence.

"Percutaneous endoscopic placement of a gastrostomy feeding tube is a good suggestion," he said. "It's a relatively safe and simple procedure that can be done at the bedside and has few risks and complications."

The oncology fellow glared at me.

"We'll keep it under consideration," Dr. Hood concluded...

"Do you know what, Mike?" Ethel said. "Dr. Hood came to visit me, and right after he left, that oncology fellow comes back and tells me one of the student doctors has access to my medical records and asks whether I was aware of this.

"I didn't know who he meant at first, then I thought, 'Maybe he's talking about Mike?'...

"I told him 'Yes, and he's been a great help to me...

"And that, in fact, *he's already a doctor - he has his PhD...*"

"Mike, Dr. Hines came by after Dr. Hood. He offered to discharge me from the hospital if I felt like I was better...

"I'm anxious to leave - But I don't want to go until the pain is under control...

"I think I'm alright - But I don't want to have to come back again."

I smiled, and lifted myself out of the chair.

"I don't want you to have to come back here, either, Ethel."

I knelt and kissed her.

"Who knows?" I said. "We'll stay optimistic."

She looked at me - Smiling as she followed my steps to the door...

CHAPTER FORTY-SIX

That evening Ethel and I sat in the darkened wardroom.

"A friend and I have the same birthday," I said. "I got him one of my favorite books - *Narcissus and Goldmund* by Hermann Hesse. Have I ever told you about it, Ethel?"

"No, Mike."

"It's about two young men who meet in a cloister. Narcissus is a born intellectual, destined for a life of study; Goldmund was put there by a cruel father to atone for his mother's sins.

"Narcissus recognizes Goldmund wasn't meant for a life of solitude - he was meant for adventure - and helps him find the courage to journey outside the cloister's walls.

"Ultimately, they meet again.

"Goldmund falls off a horse, and is brought back to the cloister near death.

"In his dying breath he says to his friend, 'I'm going back - Back to my mother.'

"Then he says, 'But what shall become of you? - You who has no mother.'

"The story ends something like, 'And Narcissus stood pierced to the heart by his friend's dying words...'

"I see it as now Narcissus has to make his own journey into the realm of the heart. It makes me think of Dr. Brand and me - I saw him with a book by Hesse about a month ago. 'Oh, one of the students gave it to me,' he says - Like it doesn't mean anything to him - He's not reading it because he enjoys it - Just another intellectual exercise...

"Still, it makes me wonder - Where do we go - Dr. Brand and me - To learn to love?"

In the dimly lit room Ethel's eyes peered into mine...

CHAPTER FORTY-SEVEN

"So I'm on my way to the cafeteria," I said, "and I'm in a big hurry because - I don't know, I guess people are just walking too slow - And I'm bumping into one person after another all the way there.

"Finally, just as I'm about to go in, I bump into the wrong guy...

"He follows me into the cafeteria.

"'I bet'chu wanna be punched right in the mouth,' he says..."

"And what did you say, Mike?" Ethel said.

"I told him, 'I'm sorry. I'm always bumping into people.'"

"And then what did he say?"

"He said, 'That's alright', and walked off."

Ethel was quiet.

"And you know what else happened, Ethel?... I was on my way to the hospital from the parking lot, and I was in another hurry. I banged my leg into the bumper of a parked car, and ripped a hole in my brand new dress pants!"

I could envision her smiling.

"Can you believe it, Ethel? I'm having really bad luck."

"You know, I was listening to a talk show the other day," she said. "They were interviewing a child psychologist about what to do when children are upset -

"She was saying how she's found that putting them in front of one of those inflatable blow-up clowns, and coaxing them to hit it, really helps them take out their aggressions..."

"So that's what you think it is - Why I bump into people and rip my clothes on things - I'm taking out my aggressions! Gosh, Ethel, I thought it was just because I'm clumsy!"

"I don't think so, Mike..."

"You know, Mike, I always thought I could keep it so people didn't get to me. 'No matter what,' I told myself, 'I wasn't going to let what anybody else said or did bother me. They weren't going to ruin my day. No way. Uh-uh'...

"But I realize now, that over the last several years they had gotten to me - And made me a miserable person - And it's only been the past couple of months that I've gotten myself out of that..."

CHAPTER FORTY-EIGHT

Saturday was my birthday.

I got up early, thinking I would study in the morning, then go over to Ethel's with cake and drinks in the afternoon.

The phone rang.

"Hi, Mike," Ethel said. "I just called to tell you I coughed up a teaspoon of blood this morning, and I'm going in to the hospital. I'll talk to you later. Bye."

She hung up.

Her voice had that excited, pleasant tone it gets whenever something bad happens.

I hesitated.

Maybe I should meet her at the hospital.

I looked at my books.

"It's just thrush," I told myself. "They'll probably make her wait in the holding area all day, then send her home with some Mycelex. I have work to do..."

There was a drizzle in the air as I made my way from the parking structure to the hospital entrance.

I strolled in wearing my short white jacket and carrying a couple grocery bags.

I walked to the holding area -

Ethel wasn't there.

I wandered through the waiting room -

No sign of her.

Slowly I edged towards the emergency room -

The doors slid open.

There was Ethel -

Sitting bolt upright in a stretcher -
Ashen gray - Features sunken -
A basin full of blood alongside of her.
Her mother sat weeping at her side - Panting, and heaving and
struggling for breath.
Ethel called to me.
"Mike... Mike..." she said. "Help Momma..."

I turned to Mrs. Small.
"What happened?!"
She just raised a hand and shook her head - Her lungs too
congested to speak.
I looked back and forth between them.
"I've got to find out what's been done," I said.
I went to the nursing station.
"Hi, I'm a friend of Ms. James'. What's going on with her?"
"She had a massive GI bleed when one of the medical students
tried to insert a nasogastric tube," said the charge nurse. "We're
waiting for her to go up the MICU [Medical Intensive Care Unit].
They told us a few hours ago that a bed was ready for her, but they
were waiting for her lab work before sending her up there."
"What's the hold up?"
"The lab says they didn't get adequate blood samples. We sent
specimens to them twice already. The first time they said the samples
got lost, and I think the second time they told us the blood was
clotted.
"The intern taking care of her is over there."
She pointed to a handsome Indian resident.
"Pardon," I said. "I'm a friend of Ms. James. The lab says it
needs more blood."
"Oh, yeah," he said.
Without hesitation, he lifted Ethel's gown above her waist,
exposing her -
Neither I nor Ethel intervened as he collected blood from an IV
in her thigh...

"Here," he said. "Give this to the nurse."
"That's okay. I'll take it to the lab myself..."
I delivered the specimens, then called to the MICU.
"We've been waiting for her," the resident said. "It's been a little
hectic here, so I haven't had time to check on her, but I'll be down
there soon..."
I went back to Mrs. Small -

"Ethel is going to be okay," I said. "Now it's your turn."

I took her to the Asthma unit, where she was immediately treated with face mask and inhalers...

The MICU resident was a perky, red-haired woman, who soared through the emergency room.

She shuffled through the ER papers.

"Everything looks in order!" she said. "Let's get her to the floor! You want to help me transport her to the unit?..."

Just as we were making our way through the sliding doors, Mrs. Small was being moved in on another gurney.

The passing stretchers slowed and halted -

Just long enough for mother and daughter to embrace...

At the MICU several units of blood had already been delivered, along with Ethel's previous record.

The MICU resident looked at the old chart.

"What?!" she cried. "There are DNR [Do Not Resuscitate] orders written for her!"

She looked up in dismay.

"That means she has no business being here!"

She cradled the heavy charts in her arms, and ran off the unit.

I hesitated.

DNR orders meant no life-sustaining measures - Not even transfusions. If she was going to get those transfusions the orders would have to be reversed -

But if we reversed them and Ethel got worse, the MICU team would be obligated to perform life-saving measures -

If we waited, though, she could bleed again - This time terminally.

I paced back and forth, playing all the possible scenarios over and over in my head.

Then, the buzz left me -

Oh, shit. She bled because the Baritol burned a hole in her stomach. That can be fixed. We'll get her off the Baritol and put her on something else - She needs a transfusion now!

I went into the room.

"Ethel. There's something we have to discuss. When you were first diagnosed, you signed Do Not Resuscitate orders..."

"Yes," she said. "They told me that if I didn't I might have to be kept alive on machines. I didn't want to be a burden to anyone..."

"I understand - The thing is, those orders takes you out of the realm of what they can do for you here.

126

"In your case, you've had a GI hemorrhage and lost a lot of blood. A transfusion can correct that, but under the DNR orders it's seen as a life-prolonging measure, and the doctors here can't legally write for it."

"Oh... Well, if it's for a transfusion, I think that's alright...."

We reversed the DNR orders, and transfusions were begun - Soon there was life in her face again.

"Mike, when I first saw you coming into the emergency room I thought you had something in your hands - Like you were carrying some brown paper bags with you."

"Yes, Ethel," I mumbled. "I bought some cake and cookies on the way over..."

I looked at the floor.

"It's my birthday."

She smiled.

"Oh, happy birthday, Mike...

"For some reason I thought your birthday was on Tuesday. Yeah, happy birthday...

"I told Momma I was planning on going shopping today so I could find an inflatable punching bag for you."

Then, with an amused expression, she looked down at the lines and wires coiled around her.

"That was before all this happened..."

CHAPTER FORTY-NINE

I brought a copy of *Narcissus and Goldmund* to the hospital, thinking I would read to Ethel -

But she spent the day pleasantly resting, and I read to myself.

Janet looked over my shoulder -

"'The struggle between the flesh and the spirit,'" she read. *"What's it about?"*

I told her about the two characters.

"Which one do you identify with?"

"Both," I lied.

She smiled, her eyes directed downward...

I was getting ready to leave when Dr. Webster came in through the back corridor -

He had been the Dean of Students at the Office of Student Affairs, and Ethel's superior for twenty years.

We'd met at a gathering just before I left for the NIH.

"I'm afraid I'll forget everything I've learned," I'd confided, "and lose all my clinical skills."

"Just like riding a bicycle," he'd said expansively. *"You never forget...."*

He entered Ethel's room.

I watched as she lifted her long graceful arms to embrace him.

"Are you following the patient?"

It was one of Dr. Webster's residents.

"Dr. Webster has especially requested she be transferred to his service when she gets out of the MICU," he said. "We'll follow her here, and keep checking on her till she comes to the floor."

"Thank God," I thought. "We're home..."

CHAPTER FIFTY

I went out the next evening, and didn't get back till late -

I thought about visiting Ethel, but was sure Dr. Webster was taking good care of her.

Shoniah called -

"Dr. Webster talked to Momma," she said. "He told her she didn't have too long to live."

"What did he mean, Shoniah?! - 'Didn't have too long to live.' - Was he talking weeks, months - Hours, days?!"

"It seemed like he meant *days* - Maybe just a couple...

"He says they saw air in her abdomen, and she has a tear in her stomach. They offered to do surgery, but we told them we didn't want any."

I stared at the books on my desk.

"Shoniah, I have to prepare for an EEG conference tomorrow," I said. "I'll be there in a couple hours."

I hung up the phone.

"Oh, Mike. What's the matter with you?! Ethel's just been told she has just two days to live, and you're worried about reading EEGs!

"Where is your heart?!"

I pushed the books aside, and threw on my white jacket...

The GI service had performed endoscopy on Ethel earlier in the day, and found an ulcer, described as probably NSAID-induced.

An X-ray performed after, showed air under the diaphragm, suggesting a perforation of the bowel.

If this were the case, then left untreated, the contents of her stomach would slowly spill into her abdominal cavity, resulting in sepsis and death...

I crept into the room.

Ethel, her eyes shut, lay reclining and smiling in bed.

"So, you finally got here, Mike," she said in a reassuring tone.

"Sorry I didn't come earlier, Ethel. I went out with a friend last night, and today was kept late on rounds."

She became quiet - Her eyes downcast.

"I told Mike about what Dr. Webster said," Shoniah said.

"Did I not do the right thing, Mike?"

There was a change in her voice - More excited - Unnerved.

"We'll talk to the doctor's about it tomorrow, Ethel," I said. "How do you feel about the possibility of surgery?"

"I really don't think I'm strong enough..."

"Momma, do you want me to bring you any food?" Shoniah said.

"I wanted steak earlier. Mike, can I eat that?"

"I don't know, Ethel. What did your doctor's say?"

"They said she could eat anything she wants," Shoniah responded.

The woman has a perforation, and they're telling her she can eat whatever she wants?! It doesn't make sense!

"Well, I guess if they said she could eat anything, she can eat anything," I said lamely.

Ethel closed her eyes.

"Shoniah! Go home!"

Her tone was severe and abrupt - Even she seemed aware of it.

"Go home," she repeated softly.

Shoniah turned and walked obediently to the door.

Her hand on the knob, she turned and looked back.

Then, faster than I could follow, she was at her mother's side -

The contents of her bags spilling to the floor, as the two kissed, and then again...

Without another word, Shoniah collected her things and left.

Ethel lay drifting in and out.

"I want pancakes!" she blurted.

Her words were unprompted -

Were the radiologists right? I thought. Did she have a perforation? Was she slipping away into sepsis?

I scanned her abdomen -

The energy was broad and diffuse, and expanded like a bubble against my arm -

My scalp began to tingle, and the bones of my skull breathed in and out around my eyes...

At around midnight Janet peeked into the room.

"What's going on?" she whispered.

"Has Shoniah spoken to you yet?"

"No. I just got here."

"We better talk..."

I took her to the waiting room.

"We can't know for sure," I said. "But we've got to prepare ourselves for the worst..."

Janet looked at me blankly for a moment - Then turned her head away and began to weep - Her shoulders so hunched and body curled that she had trouble getting out of the chair where she was sitting.

"I'm okay... I'm okay..." she insisted.

I followed her back to her sister's room.

"I'll stay with her tonight," she said.

"Good. Then I'm going home...

"If for any reason she wakes up and asks for me, call me at home immediately!

"I don't want her to feel abandoned!..."

The next morning I met Janet outside Ethel's room.

"Morning, Janet. How was last night? Did Ethel ask for me?"

"Yes, Mike. She asked where you were."

"Oh, no!" I cried.

"Wait a minute, Mike - Let me finish," she said, smiling. "I said, 'Mike went home to get some rest, and he'll be back tomorrow.'

"Then, she said, 'Okay,' laid her head down, and went back to sleep."

"Did she say anything else?"

"We talked a little bit - 'I can't give up!' she told me. 'I want to be there for my grandson growing. I want to see my grandchild on the way. I have to go on fighting...'"

CHAPTER FIFTY-ONE

I went to the Oncology office looking Dr. Hood.

But the door was locked, and I decided to go back upstairs.

Then, in the glass-enclosed stairwell, I saw Dr. Brand making his way to the hospital entrance.

Wearing a thinly insulated gray jacket, bundled against the cold, he was pleasantly engaged in conversation with a woman walking along side of him.

I raced up the steps to meet him on the fifth floor...

"Hey there," he said, stepping off of the elevator. "What's going on, Mike?"

"Ethel's back in the hospital," I said. "She's in the MICU.

"I need your advice on something..."

We walked to his office.

"She came in on Saturday," I said, still out of breath, "with a GI bleed, probably Baritol induced. They were able to stabilize her with transfusions, but an abdominal X-ray shows air under the diaphragm."

"Oh, gosh," he said, *changing into his white coat.*

"The GI service offered her surgery, but she and her daughter refused, saying she was too weak -

"I think I can get them to change their minds, though..."

Ethel was barely conscious when we entered the room.

Seeing Dr. Brand, though, a contented smile stretched across her features -

"Hi, Dr. Brand... I'm fine... They won't let me... They won't let me... They won't let me sit."

"No? Well, we can probably get you a chair. Don't get upset. You're in the MICU. They have lots of monitors and IVs and things, but they don't have little things like chairs."

He looked about uncertain - Like a small boy caught in a position of overwhelming responsibility.

Ethel's head leaned to the right, as she struggled to maintain consciousness.

"Lie back, Ms. James!" he said, pushing her head back. "You don't have to pull your head forward that way!"

"Is it... Is it... Is it raining out?" she asked.

"No," he said curtly. "It's a nice, sunny day. We could open the shutters if you'd like to look outside."

I went to the window, but couldn't find a knob.

"Here, Mike. You need a special key to open that thing."

He stepped in front of me and opened them himself.

Returning to the bedside, he took out his stethoscope, laid it on her abdomen, sat curled up on a stool, and listened.

Dr. Kumar from the GI service walked in with his resident.

"Look!" he said. "She is smiling for the first time!"

Dr. Brand looked up.

"You guys from GI?" he said. "She feels a little tight..."

Dr. Kumar and the resident tip-toed out...

Dr. Brand got up and sheepishly took a few steps back.

"Well, we're gonna go outside and talk to some of these doctors. I'll be back to see you later."

I followed him out.

"It looks like she's dying, Mike. I think comfort measures are the best we can offer at this point."

"Dr. Brand, tell me something - *What is the measure?* - I mean, *what are we basing this on?* Besides her anemia and hypoalbuminemia, her labs are okay - She's got an iatrogenically-induced ulcer, and bled a couple of times, but that can be corrected..."

"Her abdomen feels tight, though, Mike!" he interrupted, "and there's no active bowel sounds! It could be from iatrogenic causes, as you say, but it could also be expansion of her tumor - When they took her to the OR and opened her up and got in there, they could find tumor everywhere. You could try aggressive measures and buy her a little time, but at the same time you might kill her!

"The way I see it, we've given her another six months she wouldn't have otherwise had, and now it's time to say 'Enough.'

"I try to approach these things philosophically, saying, 'If this were me, how would I like this handled? - I have this diagnosis - I've

134

*had six months to prepare - Now I'm ready to go out - And I don't
want a lot of life-saving measures because they're just more harm
than they're worth."'*

"Dr. Brand, pardon me for taking your time, but let me ask you
this - What if you approached this from Ethel's philosophical point of
view? She's reacted to all of this like she's been sick, and treated the
last six months as a time of healing. She didn't want to hear
prognoses - She wanted to focus her energies on getting well. Now
it's thrust upon her that she's going to die and has only days to live.
For her this is something sudden. With that in mind, should
measures be taken so she could possibly have a couple of weeks - *or
just a week!* - to prepare herself for death?"

His gray-blue eyes had been darting back and forth between
each of mine -

Now they fixed on me, and suddenly became red and glazed
over -

Then, an instant later, his whole body convulsed and recoiled, as
though sustaining a blow to the chest -

He stood bent over, supporting himself with his hands against
his thighs; breathing violently through his nostrils; and struggling to
make his way back to me -

*"Mike! You might buy her a few weeks, but she's very fragile, so
you also might kill her!"*

*"And, then, who knows," he said, his voice raspy. "Some people
never come to terms with dying, and so all you've wound up doing for
them is giving them a couple of weeks of false hope.*

*"I have an aunt who recently passed. Strong person - just like
her. She had stomach cancer - It was very fast. Her husband smoked,
drank - She didn't do any of that. Sixty-five - Boom! - She was gone."*

*"Now, I know it's difficult for you because you're her friend,"
and looked away for the first time, "but I think comfort care
measures are the best we can do at this point...*

*"People know when they're gonna die. There are the Kubler-
Ross stages - denial and all that - But usually people know..."*

"That's the best I can tell you," he concluded, assuming his
familiar, subdued tone. "Sorry, Mike."

I nodded, and watched him walk away...

"I don't know what I could have said," I told Cynthia that
evening.

*"I know exactly what you said!" she responded. "To guys like
him it's all about death! - It's about control! And if you're not getting
healthy their way, then they just want you to check out and get ready*

to die! - And that's not at all what their patients are thinking. They haven't a clue that to their patients it's all about life!"

"That kind of realization is enough to make you want to go out and hang yourself!" she continued.. "I would! Your innocent remark really socked him. If you used the same words to him that you just told me, then, basically, you just told him that everything he's done his whole life - or, at least, his entire professional career where cases like Ethel's are concerned - was completely wrong!..."

CHAPTER FIFTY-TWO

Muffled voices trailed through the corridor as I made my way to the MICU that evening -

"But they said they would give me something... give me something... to stop the hurting... stop the hurting..."

"We have already given you the medications the doctor's prescribed," a soft voice responded.

I turned the corner -

Ethel was pleading with a male nurse.

"But they said they would give me something... to stop the hurting... stop the hurting..."

I stepped into the room -

"What's the matter, Ethel?"

"Mike... Mike... They said they would give me something... to stop the hurting..."

"Where is it hurting, Ethel?"

"All over my stomach... my stomach..."

"Let's see what we can do."

I scanned her abdomen - The energy pulled my hand closer until it came to rest against her skin, and held me there.

I looked up, uncomfortable being in the hospital this way - The nurse coming and going every few minutes.

I knelt on the floor, curled my arm around her, and pulled her close to me.

Her breathing became less labored.

"Thank you, Mike. I feel better... feel better..."

I laid her down, and she drifted off to sleep.

In the hallway the male nurse stood in my path.

I tensed, preparing myself for what he might say.

He smiled, full and radiant.
"Thank you, Mike," he said...

CHAPTER FIFTY-THREE

Wednesday, February 4, 1998

Shoniah and I stood outside her mother's room.

"May I ask you a question?" I said. "Are your prepared for your mother's death?"

"Yes. Yes, I am," she responded. "The way I see it, the spirit just goes on and on...

"The only thing I'm interested in, is I don't want her to suffer..."

Ethel lifted her head and smiled beseechingly when she saw me entering the room.

"Mike... Mike... Will you... Will you... Will you do something for me?... Help me sit... Help me sit... Help me sit up in bed... Will you help me? Will you please?"

"Sure, Ethel. Just give me a second to ask the nurses if it's okay..."

"No!.. No!... Not the nurses! Don't ask the nurses! Not the nurses!"

She burst out crying.

"Mike... Mike... Have I ever... Have I ever... Have I ever been mean to you?... Have I ever been mean? Have I ever been mean to you?"

"No, Ethel. Of course not. Never."

"These nurses here been calling me 'mean.' They say I'm mean. They say I'm mean, Mike."

Tears fell from her eyes.

"They're mean. They're mean, Mike. They won't help me. They won't let me get in a comfortable position. They're mean. They make

me poop all over myself. They won't let me go to the bathroom. They say I have to poop on myself.

"Then, when they come to clean it, they use a wash cloth soaked in ice cold water! Who would do that?! Who would do another person that way?!"

Out of the corner of my eye I caught sight of Shoniah - Her face reddened and eyes glazed over, till a look of anguish ripped her features, and she turned her head away.

"I can't take much more of this! Uh, uh! I can't take much more of this! I have to boo... I have to boo-boo... I have to boo-boo. I can't use the toilet! Why won't they... Why won't they... Why won't they... Mike... Please... Please... I've never... I've never... I've never done anything to you. Please. Please. Help me. Won't you help me? Please help me. Won't you please?!"

Tears welled up in my eyes -

But, also, a feeling of inner strength, as energy beamed from my head.

"Of course, I'll help you, Ethel. Here. Let me sit you up in bed... Then we'll move one leg to the side... Good. Now, the other... Shoniah will help us, okay?..."

Ethel guided us -

"Okay... No... Okay... No... Okay..."

I went to face her -

"Here, Ethel, put your arms around my shoulders... That's it. I'm going to help pull you up. Are you ready?... Okay, here we go... One - Two - Three."

Ethel breathed a sigh of relief -

"Oh, thank you, Jesus, thank you. Lordy, lordy. Mike, you don't know how good that feels. Oh, thank you. Thank you..."

CHAPTER FIFTY-FOUR

An attractive ICU nurse came into the room with an Italian ice for Ethel.

"I thought it would be good for her," she said, "because she's only had normal saline for days and her sugar would be diluted."

"Oh, yes," I responded. "She loves Italian ices. Watermelon. That's her favorite."

I took the ice, and began feeding Ethel.

The nurse made a face, then turned and left the room.

"I hope she didn't feel insulted," I said.

Shoniah shrugged her shoulders...

A few minutes later the nurse was back.

"Visiting hours are over," she said. "You're going to have to leave the room now."

I stood my ground.

"You can come back in an hour," she added...

When we returned, the nurse was repositioning Ethel -

"Are you alright? Let's move just a little more... I don't know how you feel, but I'm sure it isn't very good... Do you want to rest more?... Give me your hand. No, give me your hand, dear. I know you're not very comfortable. Just a little bit more... What did you say? I couldn't hear you. I'm sorry Mrs. James, I didn't hear what you said..."

She was very competent (as well as lithe and beautiful), but had a snappy way about her.

"All that woman ever does is yap at you!" I cried after she'd left. "In a past life she must have been one of those little dogs that's always biting at your heels - *Yap, yap, yap, yap, yap!*"

An ethereal voice rose up and spoke to me from all four corners of the room -

"*Mike, when I get out of here, I'm gonna take you over my knee and give you a spanking.*"

"What?!"

I whipped my head around.

Ethel, her eyes closed, sat smiling -

Displaying sparkling pearl white teeth...

CHAPTER FIFTY-FIVE

Dr. Kumar smiled at me as he entered the MICU.

"I saw you the other day with Dr. Brand, right?" he said. "Are you a friend of Mrs. James?... What do you think about the way she is doing?"

"Well, I understand that surgery..."

"We feel that comfort measures are best at this time," he interrupted. "Although many interventions could have been tried, we talked to Mrs. James and her daughter and decided that recuperation in the hospital with a two-foot long scar down the middle of your belly wasn't the best way to spend the last days of your life. The plan now is to transfer her to the ward, then let her go home. Do you have any concerns or questions?"

"Yes, I do. What if she bleeds again? What then?"

"That's fine. If it's a fast bleed, she will go into a coma. If it's a slow bleeder, then hopefully the family will know what to do."

I stared at him blankly.

"I'm sorry you had to see all this with your friend," he said, "but you will see a lot more in the years to follow..."

"It seemed to leave me so quick."

I'd been sitting next to her.

"What's that, Ethel?" I said. "I wasn't listening - Were you talking about last night? - That I left too quick?..."

"No - 'It' - It seemed to leave me so quick. I was feeling fine, then it all left me so quick... Quick... Quick... It left me so quick... Why did it leave so quick?... So quick... Quick."

"Ethel, your body is very fragile. When we left the hospital last week, I was hopeful like you. I thought we had the pain under control, and we could focus on your nutrition, and, if need be, go for the G-tube.

"But an ulcer developed - And now it could be that it's..."

"Burst?" she said, more present than any time since Dr. Webster's pronouncement.

"Yes - Perforated - 'Burst' - It came about because of everything you've been through."

"What's gonna happen now, Mike?"

"Now, we're going to make sure you're comfortable. The opinion is that you're not going to get better. There's no way of knowing how long. It might be days or weeks. We can't know for sure."

"Where should I go now, Mike? Where should I go? Should I go home? Is that what I should do? Should I go home now? Home? Is that right?"

"I just spoke to Dr. Kumar. He said he wanted you here during the night, then we'll go home tomorrow. That's the plan..."

Shoniah came into the room.

"Mike, can you come out for a minute... I have the social worker here, and we're talking about what to do with Momma."

The social worker was a dull-looking woman with smeared blue-gray irises.

"The plan is to send her to The Marymount hospice," she announced through half-closed eyes.

"What?!" I said. "I just got through telling her she's going home!..."

"According to my knowledge, the plan is to send her to hospice."

"But I just spoke to Dr. Kumar - He said the plan was to send her home with a PCA pump..."

"I don't think that's possible - They don't let patients have PCA pumps at home. That's something they're experts at over at hospice."

She moved closer, and whispered as though confiding.

"You see, the problem here is the family didn't make any definite arrangements in advance, and now they don't know what they want to do. Do you know how long they've been planning this?"

"Well, the precipitating event happened all of a sudden."

"Hmmf," she said, then turned and scoffed off.

She returned a minute later.

"Dr. Kumar agrees with the current planning for Mrs. James," she announced.

"And what's that?" I said.

"That she be transferred to another hospital."

"Well, did you ask him about what I told you?"

"No, I didn't ask him that."

"Well, why not?!"

"I didn't think of it. If you want, you can talk to him... He's in the conference room."

I pulled open the door, and marched in the direction of the delicately built Indian physician.

"I just wanted to make sure of I heard you right - Did you say it was possible for Ms. James to go home with a PCA pump?"

He hesitated.

"I think the plans with the social worker are alright," he said.

A sheepish look graced his features.

I didn't have the heart to ask him anything more...

CHAPTER FIFTY-SIX

A big heavyset man stood over the bed when I went back to Ethel's room.

Shoniah was next to him, and had his same coloring and complexion.

"Hi, Mike," she said. "This is my dad."

"Nice to meet you," I said.

He nodded. His expression was overly serious - Like a child who needs to prove something.

Then he lowered his head till it nearly touched Ethel's.

"Be strong!" he said. "Don't stray! Be faithful!..."

A pained expression gripped her features -

She tightened her lids over her eyes and nodded, unable to pull away.

"Remember!..."

Finally, he straightened, and abruptly walked to the door.

In the narrow confines of the room we were pressed together, and I stood in his way.

"What do I call you besides 'Dad'?" I said.

"Samuel," Shoniah responded.

"Oh." I looked up, affected. "Like your grandson."

A bright good-natured expression stretched across his features, and he smiled and laughed heartily...

CHAPTER FIFTY-SEVEN

I gaze at the woman lying in the bed,
Eyes barely open,
Somewhere between limbo and decay.
Suffering.
Something we all do.
Ah, but beautiful suffering,
Something there that extends beyond self,
Opens an invisible doorway,
And let's each other in...

Ethel awoke, and called to me faintly.
"Are you writing, Mike?"
I stood at the foot of the bed, and peeped up from my papers,
like a child caught making a gift for a parent, not wanting her to see.
"Yes." I said. "I am."
"Oh," she said, an enticing smile on her lips.
"I'll read you what I've written," I said, having no intent to do
so.
"Okay, Mike."
She continued to smile - And drifted back to sleep...

CHAPTER FIFTY-EIGHT

Brian (the MD/PhD student) greeted me in the hallway.

"Hey," he said. "What service are you on this month?"

"I'm here because Ethel was recently admitted."

"Oh, yeah." He straightened his tall, gangly frame. "How's she doin'?"

"She had a GI bleed," I said.

He furrowed his brow in what looked like a well-practiced troubled expression.

"I'm disappointed," he said. "I hoped she'd respond better to the things we did for her..."

CHAPTER FIFTY-NINE

Ethel hadn't eaten in two days.

Shoniah brought some food from home, and Janet went to feed her.

"I can do it," Ethel insisted.

She picked up the spoon and fork, but held them like she didn't know how to - Gripping them as though her hands had been transformed into a pair of useless claws.

I looked on, certain she would breakdown and weep.

But the good-natured expression never left her, even as she labored in vain with the utensils.

"Let Mike do it!" Janet pleaded.

"Yeah, Mom!" Shoniah said.

An embarrassed smile graced Ethel's features - The utensils still dangling from her hands.

"Oh, alright."

She shook her head, still smiling.

"You win," she laughed.

Janet smiled and merrily clasped Ethel's hands.

"You win..."

I took the utensils.

"You better be careful," I said. "I've had friends who've told me they wouldn't trust me with their children because they'd be afraid I'd let them starve."

"Why's that?" Shoniah said.

"Because I'd only feed them when and what they wanted to eat."

Ethel withdrew.

Ethel prized her independence, and here I was comparing her to a baby...

She dutifully took what I fed her.
"If her stomach is perforated," I thought, "then feeding her could be making things worse."
I stared down at the meal -
It looked and smelled appetizing -
As though lovingly prepared...

CHAPTER SIXTY

During the night Ethel was moved to a ward room on the sixth floor.

Mr. Small arrived mid-morning.

"Where's Mrs. Small?" I said.

"I couldn't bring her," he said. "Her lungs are bad..."

Ethel was barely conscious.

I glimpsed over at Mr. Small, and caught a worried look.

Without a word, he got up and walked to the door.

"Something the matter, Mr. Small?" I said.

He pulled back, startled.

"No. No. Nothing's a matter."

He left the room...

There was a knock on the door, and a professionally dressed woman entered.

"Hi, I'm looking for Shoniah. My name is Sheryl. I'm a representative from The Marymount hospice. I just had to get you to sign a few forms before we transport your mother."

Shoniah turned to me.

"You want to come, Mike?"

Sheryl took us to another room -

She explained the arrangements -

I was watching Shoniah, and wasn't listening...

Dr. Brand appeared walking towards us - His movements so finely tuned he seemed to glide.

"Hi, Mike. How are you doing?"

He held out his hand -

To my surprise, it was cold and clammy.

"Just fine, Dr. Brand. *How are you?*"

I searched his eyes.

"Fine, Mike."

He avoided my glance.

I turned to Shoniah.

"By the way," I said, "this is Ethel's daughter..."

He stepped in front of me, smiling and vigorously shaking her hand -

"Hi, I'm Dr. Brand. Nice to meet you..."

An awkward silence followed.

"Well, I just spoke to her," he said. "I just wanted to let you know we had a nice conversation."

"That's great..."

But before I could finish, he'd turned and walked away.

"What did he do that for?" I thought. "Did he feel like he had to?"

But watching him walk off I felt more concerned for him than I did for Ethel...

I was sitting next to Ethel when Dr. Webster and his team collected at the doorway.

"Good morning," he said.

I got up from my chair, and he and the members of his team congregated around Ethel.

"How's everyone doin'? How you feelin', Ethel?... That's good... No, if it was a perforation we would have seen something by now. Okay, we'll come back a little later. See y'all."

He walked out.

Wait a minute! I thought. If she doesn't have a perforation, what are we going to hospice for?!

Dr. Webster was still in the hallway talking to Shoniah.

I decided to approach him with my concerns -

But as soon as I took a step in his direction, he scooted past her and walked away.

I sat dumbfounded.

"What's up, Mike?" Shoniah said.

"I don't understand - Arrangements were made to go to hospice because your mother had a perforation, and there was nothing else we could do for her.

"Now we're told she doesn't have a perforation, yet the plan remains the same - It doesn't make sense."

Just then, I saw Dr. Hood at the nurse's station. I waited for him to come and visit Ethel, but his team was dispersing and he was walking the other way.

"Shoniah, I'll be right back. I want to catch Dr. Hood..."

I ran through the hallways.

"Dr. Hood... Dr. Hood..."

He turned.

"Oh, hi, Mike. I was just going to the MICU to see Ethel. How is she?"

"She was transferred to the wards last night."

"What's the plan with her?"

"They're getting ready to send her to The Marymount hospice..."

We made our way back to Ethel's room.

"I don't understand it," I said. "If perforation is out of the picture, why are we still going to hospice?..."

He listened in silence.

"Dr. Hood, what do you think we should do?"

"I think treating her at Claude Ray might be just as comfortable as a hospice setting. If we could get her an isolation room, I think that would be optimal..."

Entering the room he knelt beside her.

"Ethel. It's Bryce. How are you?..."

Behind me I heard the sound of something metal, and saw two EMTs (Emergency Medical Transport personnel) preparing a stretcher.

Dr. Hood stood in front of me.

"Keep in contact with me," he said. "Let me know where they take her."

"Dr. Hood, tell me - If we could do anything at this moment, what would be the best thing?"

The EMTs guided their stretcher past us.

"Should we buck the system?!"

He stood his ground.

"I think it will be okay, Mike. We'll go with the current plan..."

CHAPTER SIXTY-ONE

The EMTs were two muscularly built African American men.

I thought they would be rough with Ethel -

But the two were so skillful that their transfer from bed to gurney left even Ethel smiling.

"You're good!" she said.

I followed them to the ambulance -

I expected them to by cynical - Wonder what a "white-boy" was so worried about a black woman for.

One turned.

"You wanna ride over with us?..."

They secured her in the ambulance.

"What's she got?" the one said.

"Pancreatic cancer."

"How long she's had it?"

"She was diagnosed six months ago."

"That fast?..."

It was a cold, clear, crisp winter day, and the skies were radiant and blue.

But getting out of the ambulance the cold air blew between the buildings and left me chilled. The two men lifted Ethel out of the ambulance - Her neck and torso exposed.

They wheeled her to the admitting area, situated in a drafty corridor just outside the hospital.

"We have an admit from Claude Ray," the EMT said.

"Well, let me call and see if they're ready for her," replied the bland-looking woman at the counter.

I tucked myself in my white jacket - The cold air blowing through me.

"No," she said, "the nurses up there say the room isn't ready for her yet. You'll have to wait here."

I searched the closets for blankets, but couldn't find any.

What kind of a hospital is this?!

The EMTs grumbled between each other, then went back to the woman at the desk.

"Hey, what floor is that room supposed to be on?" the one said.

He turned to his partner.

"Com' on, let's get going..."

The room was crammed with furniture - Most had to be moved into the hallway before the stretcher could pass.

The EMTs gathered their things.

"God bless," the one said...

"How are you feeling, Ethel?" I asked.

"I'm kind of having some pain in my back. I think my last morphine dose has run out."

I went to the nursing station. There was an Asian woman behind the desk.

"Excuse me. I'm a friend of the newly admitted patient. She's having pain in her back, and needs some morphine."

"I'm sorry," the nurse responded. "No orders have been written for this patient."

No orders?! I thought. What is this?! We're not in County anymore!

"The woman has pancreatic cancer," I said. "She's got to have morphine immediately!"

"I will page the hospice doctor, Dr. Bork. Do you want to talk to him?..."

The phone rang a moment later.

"Yes, Dr. Bork. The new patient is here, and is complaining of pain... Okay, yes, we will begin an IV and give her the morphine...

"Also, there is a medical student here. Would you like to talk..."

She stopped abruptly.

"Oh... Okay... Yes... Yes..."

She hung up the receiver.

"He says he will be by to talk to *the family* this afternoon..."

Back in the room a group of nurses had encircled Ethel -

"Are you alright, Mrs. James?!... Is everything okay?!... Is there anything you'd like us to do for you?!..."

"Why are you always shouting?" Ethel said. *"Why aren't there any orders. They told us before we got here that everything would be ready. Why hasn't anything been done?..."*

"Well, what would you like us to do for you, Mrs. James?! Is there anything we can do to help?!..."

Most of the nurses retreated.

"Are you alright, Ethel?" I said.

"My back's really hurting."

"Maybe it would help to change your position."

I moved alongside her -

Just then, the last remaining nurse stepped in front of me.

"I'll do that!" she insisted.

She straddled Ethel, then yanked at her lower half.

"Oh, I've thrown my back out!" she shouted, clasping her back. "I only came from the chiropractor yesterday. I'm going to have to call again and get another adjustment..."

She dashed out.

Ethel looked at me.

"Mike, I want to get out of this place! I want to go home! Don't you think it would be better to go home?!"

I went back to the nurse's station.

A nurse's aide was standing there.

"Hello, I'd like to contact Dr. Bork."

"Well, you called him before, and he didn't want to talk to you. If he didn't want to talk to you then, I see no reason to bother him with you now."

"Please, it's important that I talk to him."

"Well, if you're not family, and he didn't want to talk to you before, I don't see any reason for calling him again."

She smiled with rosy cheeks.

"Is that okay?" she said.

I hesitated.

"No," I said. "No - It's not okay."

She flushed - Then turned and walked off.

I stood alone staring into the sterile confines of the ward.

The nurse's aide came back - This time accompanied by a stout, angry-looking woman with scaly skin rashes on her scalp and elbows.

"Okay," she barked, "what have we got here?"

"Perhaps I should have expressed myself earlier," I said. "But I didn't, and that's my fault...

"The reason we agreed to hospice was because we thought the woman in there had a perforated stomach, and there was nothing left to do.

"Just before leaving, though, we're told she probably doesn't have a perforation - And I can't help but wonder what we're doing here?..."

The nurse manager had positioned herself directly in front of me.

Tears welled-up in her eyes as she listened.

Without a word, she turned, and she and the aide floated into the distant corridors, their shoulders hunched...

"Dr. Bork has been notified."

The nurse's aide stood in the doorway.

"He said he'd be here in about an hour."

She looked at me with forlorn expression.

"Thank you," I said.

She turned, and walked away...

The members of Ethel's family percolated into the room. Shoniah and Janet brought Ethel's aunt Gerald. Mr. Small arrived - This time with Mrs. Small.

"Mike, this isn't a nice place!" Ethel said. "This isn't a nice place at all! I don't like this place! I want to go home! I think it's better to go home!"

Mrs. Small and Aunt Gerald shook their heads and spoke in muffled disapproving tones.

"You spoiled girl," Mrs. Small chided.

"Uh, huh," Aunt Gerald chimed in.

"You don't know what I'm feeling?!" Ethel responded. "Don't you understand how I feel?!..."

Dr. Bork arrived mid-afternoon.

He stood in the doorway and inspected Ethel -

"Oh, yes, I remember you," he said in a gruff manner. "You worked in the Office."

He perched himself on a stool, and addressed the family -

"Now, first, let me explain to you all how we do things in hospice. We don't use a PCA pump here - Our experience is that nervous family members turn out to be the ones pressing on the button and over sedating the patient to allay their own worries about how much their mother or daughter is suffering. That takes away from the whole point - PCA stands for *'Patient* Controlled Anesthesia'. We feel we can do a lot better job controlling the patient's pain ourselves..."

He got up and examined Ethel -

157

In the time it took for me to look away as he palpated under her gown, he'd disappeared...

From the doorway I saw him streak down the corridor.

I chased after him; Shoniah not far behind.

"Wait! Dr. Bork! There's something I have to ask you."

He stopped, and leaned heavily against the wall.

"Ethel entered hospice on the premise that she had a perforation," I said. "Today, we're told she doesn't - The equation has all changed..."

"Wait a minute!" he said in a harsh, authoritative tone. "What brought her into the hospital?!"

"She coughed up some blood, and had an episode of GI bleeding."

"And what set off the bleed?!"

"On endoscopy they found an antral ulcer."

"And why did she have an ulcer?!"

"GI thought it was caused by the Baritol she was taking for pain."

"And why was she in pain?!"

"Probably because of retroperitoneal expansion of the tumor."

"Maybe I have to try another approach of getting at this - What is her primary diagnosis?"

"Pancreatic cancer."

"There! That's what I've been trying to get you to say. Her primary problem is the cancer. That's what's behind everything that's wrong with this woman."

"Pardon me, but the opinion regarding her ulcer was that it was nonsteroidal anti-inflammatory-induced."

"Maybe the NSAIDs made them bleed, but the ulcers were pancreatic in origin!"

I looked at him blankly.

"You see she's swollen!... What's the cause of that?!"

"Hypoalbuminemia..."

"Liver failure! She's not making any albumin!"

"But she hasn't been eating well. It could be the result of malnutrition."

"And the ascites?! That's because of cancer cells spreading all over her peritoneum..."

I nearly shook my head in disbelief -

How could he make such assertions?! - With no diagnostic proof!

"The problem here is you're looking for something to treat. You see hoof prints, but you're looking for zebras.

"That's understandable - You're her friend - You're not thinking objectively."

"Dr. Bork, my problem is this - A perforated bowel I could accept as endgame - then it's time for hospice care, and to call it quits..."

"That depends on how you define 'endgame'. You think she's gonna live another six months?... Alright, then - According to the United States government, that's endgame right there. By European standards, it was endgame last September."

"But what if she has a treatable source of her altered mental status? I checked her labs before leaving the Claude Ray, and found an urine culture positive for E. coli. Maybe her symptoms could be explained by a severe urinary tract infection..."

"She doesn't have any of the symptoms - She didn't have pain over her bladder or costovertebral angles. If she actually had urosepsis, she wouldn't look like that...

"Then, if we treated the UTI, would it clear her sensorium? - Who knows? Personally, if it were me, I don't think I'd want a clear sensorium at the stage she's at now."

"The woman says to me the other night, 'It left me so quick. So quick. Why did it leave me so quick?' It makes me feel if there's a treatable cause, she'd want it treated."

"The more likely explanation for her altered mental status is the medications she's on, and frank liver failure..."

"And that could happen in just one day?" Shoniah interrupted.

"Sure could! I'm not saying that it did, but it certainly could!"

"But except for her albumin, her liver function tests have been okay," I said.

"Did you measure ammonia levels? The other labs could be fine, and she could still be in failure."

"Could we look for that?"

"There's little role for diagnostic tests in hospice. Laboratory studies usually aren't done..."

Dr. Bork went back to the room -

He talked to Ethel, and wrote for antibiotics...

CHAPTER SIXTY-TWO

Saturday, February 7, 1998

Ethel drifted off, her breathing slow and labored.

I left the hospital convinced that Dr. Bork was right - And this was liver failure - And there was nothing else to do.

At 5 AM I woke up wide awake - Sure it was because Ethel had passed.

From the doorway I stood looking in-

The movement of her chest was faint, but present.

Whatever design God has for her, I thought, He meant her to live another day.

I crept into the room.

Janet had stayed with her during the night -

A white sheet pulled over her head, she looked like an enshrouded body...

About an hour later Dr. Webster peeked in.

"Hello there. How everyone doin'?"

He walked to the bed.

"Hey sleepy head."

Ethel stirred.

"Just came by to see how you were. The ladies in the Office keep asking me about'cha. Wants to know when they can see ya. That be okay?... Well, you let me know. Everybody askin' about'cha. Want to know how you're doin'... Okay. Well, see ya later. Gotta get goin'. Doin' the two pager deal..."

Ethel looked at me.

"Hi, Mike."
I got up and knelt beside her.
"I just wanted to tell you 'hi'."
"Thank you, Ethel. So happy to see you this morning. So happy you slept well."
"Well, see y'all later." Dr. Webster left the room...

Shoniah arrived -
During the night she'd made plans to take her mother out of hospice and bring her home.
Ethel looked up at her, expecting -
"Did you bring the pineapple juice?"
"No, I didn't," Shoniah said.
Ethel began to cry.
"There weren't any stores open along the way," Shoniah argued.
"But I told you it was what I wanted!"
"Well, I'm sorry, I wanted to get here early so I didn't miss Dr. Bork..."
"I'll get it for you, Ethel," I said. "Dole pineapple juice, right?... I'll be right back..."

I brought back the juice, and sat her up so she could sip it through a straw -
Fading in and out, she didn't manage even a quarter of a cup.
Who am I fooling? I thought. She's lost so much. A week without nourishment - We'll never get her back to where she was?
She motioned -
"I'm finished now - I'm finished."
I withdrew the mostly filled cup.
I had accomplished nothing, I thought. Worse, I had made it painfully obvious how hopeless the situation was.
"Thank you, Mike. Thank you."
She closed her eyes, and licked her lips.
"That was so good..."

CHAPTER SIXTY-THREE

Dr. Bork peeked through the door.

"Are we all ready?" he said.

Dressed in jeans and an open shirt, he appeared in good spirits.

He and Shoniah worked on Ethel's discharge.

Shoniah was short and aloof, and I was afraid he'd be offended.

But he remained cordial, and thoroughly helpful...

By noon Ethel was in an ambulance bound for home.

The EMTs deposited her in a stretcher bed upstairs; an automated IV pump delivering morphine.

She slept, though her breathing was congested.

Poor thing, I thought. Probably caught a cold between ambulance rides.

Still, I was optimistic -

If her body's strong enough to mount a response to virus, maybe she's better than they give her credit for.

Then I looked down at her hands, and noticed something different -

Her nail beds were stone white.

That's funny.

Earlier in the morning I'd marveled at how red and engorged they were.

The transfusions really worked, I'd thought.

Shoniah came in behind me.

"I think she knows she's home and feels much happier here," she said. "Already she looks a lot more relaxed."

Ethel did look beautiful -

Wearing the dark blue blouse from Thanksgiving; her braided hair pulled up and held in a turquoise bow; her elegant neck sloped like a swan.

I looked around the room; hospital supplies - boxes of smocks, linens, basins - were littered everywhere.

I turned to Shoniah.

"Let's clear the room."

We cleaned and dusted -

Soon the room looked open, and full of light...

I applied warm compresses to relieve Ethel's congestion.

The hours passed -

"So this is what you're going to medical school for," a voice in my head said. *"So you can spend all your time wiping some old nigger woman's runny nose?..."*

I slapped the compress in the sink, and washed and re-warmed it...

CHAPTER SIXTY-FOUR

Shoniah came back upstairs.

"Karl and I went out and got some food from Libby's, Mike," she said. "I'll take care of Momma for a while if you want to have some."

I stared down at Ethel - still resting - and nodded to Shoniah.

Downstairs Karl was sitting on the couch.

"Aye, what's up, Mike?!" he said. *"Have something to eat! The NBA All-stars game is on!..."*

We were watching the three-point shooting when Shoniah called from upstairs.

"Mike, something's wrong with the IV pump."

"What's the matter?"

"I don't know. It keeps beeping..."

The pump flashed "NO IV ACCESS."

"How long has it been beeping this way?" I said.

"For at least several minutes," she said. "I'm going to call the home-nursing supervisor, and tell her to come over and look at it..."

The nursing supervisor pulled up in her van.

She was a heavyset woman who moved infuriatingly slowly -

"There's some malfunction," she said. "I have to take it in for repairs."

"She hasn't had any access to morphine for a couple of hours," I said. "What if she wakes up?"

"If that happens, you'll have to give her the morphine orally," she said.

I stared down at Ethel.

"Put a morphine pill under her tongue," she continued. "It will dissolve there."

She lumbered down the stairs.

"I'll try to be back soon."

From the window I watched her drive away.

God, I hope she doesn't wake up!

I turned and looked at Ethel -

Already she'd begun to stir.

She moaned -

But when she tried to move, her limbs wouldn't respond.

She looked at me puzzled, and tried to speak -

But what came out were harsh, guttural sounds I couldn't understand.

Her eyes became panic stricken, and she moaned and jerked back and forth.

"I think she's in pain, Shoniah," I said. "We better give her the morphine."

"Wait a minute, Mike," she said. "She's still too sleepy. I wonder if we're not overmedicating her. Let's give her a little more time without giving her anything."

She moaned louder, and the whole bed began to shake.

"Are you in pain, Ethel?" I said. "Is that what it is?"

She rocked frantically.

"Shoniah, I'm worried. I want to give her the morphine."

"I don't think it's pain. I think it's something else."

Ethel's terror-filled eyes stared directly into mine.

I met her gaze, and a feeling of calm swept over me -

"No, Ethel," I thought. "There's no going back to the hospital. You're staying with us now. We're going to take care of you. Whatever happens, it will be with us..."

The moans and jerking grew worse, and left me feeling like I had to do something.

"Maybe she's uncomfortable," I said. "Let's change her position in bed."

Shoniah and I struggled to sit her up -

But she just cried out louder, and looked about as though to say, "No, that isn't what I needed!"

I turned to Shoniah.

"I'm giving her the morphine."

I opened the bottle, and took out a pill.

But when I went to feed it to her, her jaws remained clamped shut.

"Ethel, I want you to take this," I said. "Open your mouth."

I tried squeezing the pill between her teeth -

It just crumbled in my fingers.

"God, what are we gonna do?!"

I ran downstairs, and crushed the pill in some water - Then ran upstairs again, and spoon-fed her the mixture -

It just spilled down her chin.

"Shoniah, I'm going to do something unpleasant... It's something I learned in Pediatrics - When an infant won't open its mouth, you cover its nostrils. I'm going to do that to your mother."

I stared down at Ethel.

"Ethel, I'm going to cover your nose. I'm sorry if it's uncomfortable."

She shrieked, and writhed underneath me.

Then, her mouth opened, and I inserted the pill...

Her features were devoid of expression now, as she pushed at the pill with her tongue.

Why is she pushing it out?

Her mouth looked dry, and I thought she might be dehydrated.

I took out the remainder of the pill, and reached for the diluted mixture -

I tried to spoon feed her, but was afraid of chipping her teeth -

"Ethel, I'm going to suck the morphine into a straw, then transfer it to your mouth."

I watched her swallow -

"Are you thirsty, Ethel? I want to give you some pineapple juice."

She swallowed the juice.

But her breathing was becoming labored, and the congestion getting worse -

Suddenly, with a surge of strength, Ethel lifted herself into a seated position, panting and struggling for breath.

I stood back and watched her -

That Ethel should have to spend her final hours like this!

"I guess this is as good as she's gonna get," Shoniah said, "and we should just keep the morphine running until she passes..."

I positioned Ethel with her head up, and went back to applying warm compresses.

Ivy and Shoniah sat across from me.

"Is Momma not able to talk 'cause she's dying?" Ivy said.

A tear formed in Ethel's eye, and rolled down her cheek.

"Ivy, please. I think your mother understands what we're saying."

Ivy stroked her mother's arm -

The gesture was well meaning, but the tactile stimulation was too much -

Ethel's attempt to tell her daughter "No" came out like a deep-pitched bark...

The nursing supervisor returned.

"When I got the pump to the repair man, he turned it on and it functioned normal," she said. *"Like nothing was ever the matter..."*

Ethel kept her eyes downcast -

There was expression in her features again, and seemed to display a calm resignation -

Sadness - But resolve.

Heartache - But, also, acceptance...

Every so often, a tear fell down her cheek -

I wiped each one away -

Wanting anything but for her to feel alone...

Within an hour, she'd drifted off.

I turned to Shoniah.

"I'm going home," I said. "I want to get my vaporizer so we can set it next to her..."

It was well past midnight, and the streets were empty.

I took the vaporizer from my closet, then turned to go back.

Today is a new day, I thought.

CHAPTER SIXTY-FIVE

Shoniah met me at the door.

"How's your mother?" I said.

"She's fine. She seems to be resting comfortably."

I went upstairs.

Ethel was breathing easily -

But there was something different about her -

She looked smaller - Shrunken - Contracted somehow?

Shoniah came in behind me.

"Mike, Mom had a bowel movement while you were gone. Will you help Karl and me change her?... Karl and I will line up on each side of the stretcher - You hold Momma's head."

Shoniah brought new linens, and she and Karl turned her.

When they uncovered her, I knew.

The sheets were stained black -

She'd had another GI bleed...

Once again it was all clear -

The stone-white nails -

The agitation when she'd awoke -

That's what she'd been trying to tell us, I thought. She'd known all along.

I looked at Shoniah and Karl, still busy changing her -

Should I tell them? I thought. Should we go to the hospital?

They laid her down -

Her arms were stiff, and flexed at her sides - And swung back and forth, and rattled.

"Is she still with us?" Shoniah said.

I reached for her pulse.

"Her heart's still beating," I said.

"I don't think she's breathing."

I put my hand over her mouth, then looked up at them, and nodded.

Karl's eyes glazed over.

"I guess it's over," he said.

Shoniah bent low and kissed her mother.

"Goodbye, Momma."

Karl followed, and the two of them left the room...

I stayed, unwilling to let go as long as I felt a pulse.

I peered into her face -

Head pulled back - Mouth gaping open - Body wasted -

"She could have been someone who died of famine in Africa," I thought...

The time passed, and I began to question what I was feeling -
Maybe it's my own pulse? I thought.

I felt our two pulses at the same time -

Mine felt smooth and steady -

Hers beat strong like a drum...

Shoniah was coming in and out of the room now -

She must be wondering what I'm doing, I thought.

I cupped Ethel's hand in both of mine -

And, to my astonishment, her pulse surged in her hand - *And grow even stronger!*

"Ethel. Your heart will always be with me..."

I put her arm down by her side.

Her hand still clung to mine.

I struggled to set it free...

CHAPTER SIXTY-SIX

Downstairs, Shoniah was making calls.

Janet arrived first; Shoniah and I accompanied her upstairs.

"Rigor mortis set in," she said under her breath. "You say she died at 1:20?... Had to be longer than that."

She shook her head, and left without another word...

The nursing supervisor came back, and drew up the death certificate...

An older, sturdy-looking man from the funeral home arrived -

"Where's the body at?" he said.

Shoniah pointed upstairs.

He hurried up the staircase with heavy steps...

Mr. and Mrs. Small arrived.

"You were here, Mike?!" Mrs. Small said tearfully. "You were with her?!..."

At the foot of the stairs she took a deep breath.

Mr. Small clung to her arm -

"Maybe we could wait for the funeral man to bring her down so you don't have to climb those steps," he said.

"That's my daughter up there!" she said. "I'll get up those steps!"

He stood along side her.

"Com'on, Mike," he said, reaching a hand to me.

I stood planted.

No! I thought. I've made my peace. I'm not going up there again!

Then Mrs. Small cried out, and I leapt up the staircase -
"I never thought it would be like this!" she said. "Hurt by someone, yes - But not this way - Not like this!...

"Ethel always had a smile for everyone she met! Always that beautiful smile no matter how bad things got for her!..."
I gazed down at her.
Wrapped warmly in white blankets, her body no longer twisted -
She looked beautiful, peaceful, and at rest...

Karl helped the funeral man bring the stretcher down the stairs -
Mr. Small and I stood outside, and watched them loaded her into the awaiting Hearst.
"The spirit is strong," he said. "But the flesh is weak..."
They drove off.
"That Friday, I knew," he said. "I knew when I sees her - I knew her time was coming."
He turned to me.
"That's why I left the way I did - I knew I had to go back home and get her mother..."
"I knew it," he said choking on the words. "I knew it was her time."
I stood staring out into the darkness.
"Mike, we want you to stay in our family. We always want you to have a place in our lives..."

In the apartment I sat for a while -
Then laid a blanket on the floor...

"I'm so happy she's still with us."
Immersed in feelings of contentment, I repeated the words over and over -
"I'm so happy she's with us..."
Suddenly I awoke to a transient vision -
Ethel's dead body falling naked on a heap of other wasted black bodies -
Mouth gaping open -
Landing with a thud, before coming to rest on top of the others...
I sat up, and began to weep -
A gnawing feeling permeated my insides, as I writhed on all fours...
More family arrived -
They'd stand over me at the passageway, then make their way to the kitchen...

In the dining room they prepared a brunch -
I stayed in the passageway, weeping.
Uncle Jack got up to go home -
He stopped at the doorway -
"You take care now, you hear?"
I lifted my head.
"You, too," I said.
He looked confused, and turned to Shoniah.
"What did he say?" he asked.
"He means 'You also'," she said.
He addressed me again -
"I know what you're going through. My wife passed six months ago. You can't know what God intends for people. Sometimes, you just have to accept His will..."

The family sat at the table.
Mr. Small called to me -
"Mike, com' on now. Food's getting cold. Come and have some brunch with the rest of us now - You hear."
I shook my head, and continued sobbing.
Shoniah rose, and came over.
"Are you alright, Mike?"
No, I said.
"Mike, you were her special friend. You took care of her. You did everything you could...
"Come on. I'm going to hold you."
She put her arms around me, and lifted me as though I were weightless...
At the table I took my place next to Mr. Small -
"Dear Father. Your son and daughter are with You again in Heaven. We thank You for Your blessings on this day, and for this good meal You have prepared.
"We are thankful..."
He held my hand firmly and gently in his -
I thought of Dr. Brand, and wished he could be with us...

At around mid-afternoon I thought it was time to go home.
I had an odd feeling as I went to say goodbye -
Smiles from family members I wasn't familiar with -
Looking at me as they knew something...

The ride back home was uneventful -

But stepping into my room, the feelings caught up with me, and the weeping and gnawing at my insides returned...

I called my friend Eric.

"Mike, I can't tell you what to do," he said. *"And no matter what, it will be the right thing...*

"But I can tell you this - If you go on this way, it will eat you alive..."

Elizabeth called -

"I just had the feeling like I should call," she said. *"How is Ethel?..."*

She listened as I recounted the night's events.

"What a gift," she said. *"For a person with a broken heart...*

"Mike, the intricacies and interweavings of the fabric of the Universe never cease to amaze me...

"Here's Ethel - In her last moments in this world - Giving you a piece of her heart - To help mend your heart...

"Mike, it was never about Ethel. It was about you! Ethel's life was over - She was going to die - It's you who gets to go on living..."

But the gnawing at my insides continued, no matter how I tried to reconcile myself with last night -

"Ethel... Ethel..."

Then, looking at the doorway, a clear filtered light entered my room -

"What's the matter, Mike?"

"Oh, I'm sorry, Ethel. I feel so bad - That I made you suffer in those final hours - I can't live with myself!"

"Oh, Mike. Don't feel bad. You did everything you could. You were only trying to help me. Oh, don't feel bad, Mike. I want you to be happy - Not sad. Oh, don't feel bad, Mike. Mike..."

CHAPTER SIXTY-SEVEN

Ethel's wake was held in a church in Sunnyside.

I arrived early, and sat in the back.

A thin, darkly discolored young man took a seat across from me, and stared uncomfortably ahead.

"You're Mike, right?" he said. "I'm Scottie - Berta's son..."

Berta had been Ethel's best friend - Heart trouble had kept her away.

"Scottie has bad SLE [Systemic Lupus Erythematosis]," Ethel had said, "and now he needs dialysis because he says his kidneys have 'shut down'...

"When he calls, we often 'compare notes' on what it's like to be sick...

"One time I told him that I was having trouble sitting on the toilet seat - Because I'd lost so much weight that I was afraid I'd fall right threw.

"And you know what he said, Mike?!" she laughed. *"That he had the same problem, too!..."*

"Scottie had recently got back together with his ex-wife," she'd confided. "He said he didn't want to, because they'd gotten divorced a couple of years ago, and he really didn't think she was right for him - *But he needed someone to take care him..."*

"You done a good job with her," he said.

He looked into the distance.

"That's right. You done a good job..."

The family arrived in a limousine, and were escorted through a special entrance to the front of the chapel.

Mr. Small saw me in the back, and motioned me to come over.

It was a cold night, and people had piled their coats in the front of the sanctuary, blocking my way.

With one hand Mr. Small gripped my arm, then lifted me over the pile.

I leaned over and kissed the dignified man...

Later, in the back of the church, I was struck by a tall, handsome African American man who looked familiar -

"Oh! Matthew!"

"That's right," he said in pleasant, soothing tones, shaking my hand. "It's me..."

I went back, and sat next to Auntie.

"That was Ethel's boyfriend," she said. "I didn't like him. He didn't treat my daughter good...

"That's right - I called her my daughter. I raised her from the time she was three, you know. She was my child."

I turned to her.

"Then I have much - much - to be grateful to you for!..."

A hand reached out from behind, and gripped me by the shoulder.

"Mike, I'm going out to the hallway to get some coffee," Uncle Jack said. "Would you like to get some with me?..."

I followed him out of the sanctuary.

"Now I want to tell you something," he said. "And that this - My wife passed six months ago, and what I found is you have to make an *adjustment* - You can't go waiting for them, 'cause they ain't never coming back. You have to make an *adjustment*. That what I learned...

"Now I'm gonna give you my phone number. You give me a call and we'll get together for dinner sometime. I've taken a strong likin' to you... A strong likin'...

"Sometime, a relationship between the races can be a good thing," he said. "A good thing..."

"I just can't understand it!" Janet said. "I can't understand any of it!... Why did she take that Baritol?! She knew it was bad for her. Why did she take it?!...

"I just know if it were me, I wouldn't have taken it - I wouldn't have done what she did!..

"Something wasn't right about her. Why did she leave that job at Midland?! She left a $40,000 a year job - With all those benefits! Why would someone do that?! I'm telling you, Mike, something wasn't right about her, and it was going on long before she came down with cancer...

"I know my day is coming. It isn't too far off. I know I'm gonna go just like she did..."

Later, Janet cried a long time in her step-brother's arms...

Samuel stood on the altar, announced the time of the funeral, and said a few words.

The congregation filtered out into the center aisle, and he and I were pushed together.

"That was a nice sermon, Samuel," I said.

"Hmm," he said, and turned his head away...

The funeral service was held the next morning.

I walked in to find the church near completely segregated -

With a small contingency of mostly white Office workers sitting on the pews on the left -

The right side completely filled by Ethel's family and friends...

The immediate family still hadn't arrived, and the funeral attendants milled about anxiously.

I went to the back of the church, and poured a glass of water.

Just then the limousine carrying the family pulled up.

Funeral attendants swarmed around Shoniah.

I cast a worried glance, and our eyes met.

"And Mike, too," she told them. "He's one of the pallbearers..."

The attendants put me at the front of the funeral procession.

As the music started, I was the first to enter the sanctuary -

But, once inside, I didn't know where to go next.

I stood in front of the casket, and looked down at Ethel -

The mortician had filled in her features, and put what looked like a painted smile on her lips -

Even in death, I thought, she had to be reassuring to everyone...

"Psst... Psst..."

A couple of young funeral attendants were smiling, gesturing to the pew in front of me.

I sat.

The rest of the pallbearers and family quickly milled into the pews on the other side.

Samuel rose to the pulpit.

"First, let's turn to page 107, and read from the second paragraph..."

We flipped from page to page.

Then, midway through the service, Samuel took in a deep breath, and smiled to the congregation.

"Now, a lot of you know that I knew Ethel from when we just kids. We were high school sweet-hearts. I remember watching her on the playground - braids in her hair - thinking, 'One day I'm gonna marry that girl'.

"And she had a brother I was just terrified of... Yeah, hi, Clyde... Whoo-wee..."

"Now if there are any members of the congregation that would like to speak, we invite you to come up now," he said. "Please try to limit your comments to two minutes."

A young woman got up and stood before the congregation.

"I'm Sheryl, a nurse's aide at Dr. Blake's office where Ethel used to work. I just wanted to say that we all miss Ethel. She was warm and pleasant, and always made the patients feel welcome..."

Shoniah addressed the congregation next.

"Hi, you all. We were late coming here this morning because I was busy composing a poem. I call the poem 'No sadness', and I'm going to read it to you now. I hope all of you will read it again later and take it into your hearts the way I think Momma did..."

I do not feel sadness for my Mother's soul
Because God took her, this I know.
The past has been a real trying time
But because of my trust in the Lord, I now have peace of mind
You see, I know my mother accepted Christ
I remember exactly when.
So at this time, I pray that you all will call on Him...

A draft blew through the sanctuary, and my body shuddered below the neck.

Samuel ascended the pulpit again -

"Now, on this day, I issue to you this challenge," he said. *"To live true to your beliefs and follow the path that God has set before you..."*

Tears of resolve formed in my eyes -

My path lay in bioenergy...

The service ended and the funeral attendants signaled us to file out.

I stood head bent, waiting for the family to pass.
Mrs. Small took my hand -
"Come on, Mike."
Mr. Small stood nodding -
We left walking together...

In the parking lot we waited to go to the cemetery.
I watched as the contingency from Midland left the church.
They piled into two cars -
Then drove back to the Office...

Heavy rains had flooded the cemetery.
Wood planks had been laid down to make a path to the burial
site - But there were only enough to reach halfway.
The attendants led me to my place at the coffin.
I stood behind Matthew -
As we marched off, I took short steps so as not to trip him...
The other pallbearers carried their weight with ease, and only I
seemed to struggle.
At the end of the planks, we began a circuitous path that criss-
crossed the field.
At the grave, we set the casket down -
The surface of the coffin gleamed in the sun, as we stood in our
mud-soaked shoes...

The other pallbearers walked back.
I turned around and saw Matthew bowed over the coffin.
I would have liked to comfort him, but thought it best he have
this time alone...

I made my way across the field -
The sky was blue and radiant -
The green grass blew vibrant with the crisp winter winds -
Everything seemed teeming with life!...

Matthew returned; his big fingers flicked at the tears in his eyes.
Family approached and tried to comfort him -
He stiffened, shook his head, and barked 'No'...

Samuel gathered the family to recite David's prayer -

"The *Lord* is *my* shep*herd*
I *shall* not *want*..."

His tone and intonation was like a rap singer -
I had the feeling of being in a team huddle -
Calling out a pre-game chant -
Before taking the field, and facing the opposition...

A pleasant appearing woman wearing sunglasses approached
me.
"Hi, I'm Linda, Samuel's wife," she said. "I wanted to ask you
how all this has affected your life?"
"'How has all this affected my life?'" I said. "Would you like a
one word answer, or should I go on for a few hours?"
"You just look like you've been affected by all this," she said.
"Just anything you want to say."
I looked at the sky.
"I loved her!" I said. "I loved her - I cherished every moment - I
love her still - I never wanted it to end!..."
She shuddered behind her sunglasses, then held herself rigid,
and nodded her head...

We drove to Auntie Belle's, and unloaded the decorations from
the funeral -
A couple of the neighborhood boys walked by, and carried off
some of the plants.
Uncle Jack was incensed -
"There ain't much worse than when you have to steal plants
from someone's funeral," he said...

The house was old and run-down - With an open sewer that ran
through the front yard, and, inside, the walls were scorched black.
I went out again and looked back -
In my mind's eye I could envision Ethel peering through the
doorway - Looking out with hope, warmth and beguiling beauty.
From homes like these, I thought. What flowers spring!...

Matthew stood next to me.
"Where are you going next year?" he said.
"I don't know." I turned and looked at him. "I don't know what
I'm doing."
"Oh, yeah," he said with knowing smile. "That's right..."

At Ethel's apartment the family had prepared a reception.

Samuel sat at the head of the table, chuckling and eating, and thoroughly enjoying his guests -

"Aye, Mike," he said, carrying a large pot to the table.

I took a small cup of gumbo, and went out...

Children played on the grass adjacent an iron fence -

Their parents greeted me as I strolled the grounds...

When I returned, Shoniah was seeing her father off -

She joined me along the fence -

"What did you think of the service?" she said.

"A little mechanical."

"Like there was something missing?"

"Yes." I turned to her. "Perhaps he was missing your mother's love..."

We looked out at the blue sky.

"I'll miss Matthew," I said.

"Yeah. I don't think I'll see him again."

"One very attractive person. At least from a distance. I think your mother really enjoyed him."

"I think it was the *challenge* more than anything else."

"Oh, I don't know," I said. "I imagine she had a good time on those trips to Louisiana."

She looked at me.

"I think I'm going to go inside and call him," she said. "Invite him over for some gumbo..."

Matthew arrived a few minutes later -

Auntie Belle was in the apartment, and he sat uncomfortable in a corner and swallowed his gumbo.

"You gonna call?" Auntie said.

"What do you care if I call?!" he snapped. "You gonna call me?!"

The meek woman fell silent.

"Alright, then! Don't be asking me, 'Am I gonna call...'"

Shoniah changed the subject, saying she had to make plans to move her mother's things into storage.

"I could help!" Matthew said. "I got a trailer! I can haul her things away!...

"Just give me a time and date! I already lost one day of work at the funeral!..."

That weekend we cleared the apartment.

I hunted through her papers for a poem she'd said she'd written about a cat that crept by her window and kept her company during the day -

I found only bills, appointments and phone numbers.

Shoniah brought me a box.

"Mike, here are some cards Momma made for her stationery business."

Designed in regal blue and gold, the cards read simply, 'Thank you'...

"What are you going to do now, Mike?" Karl said. "I mean it seemed like taking care of Ethel was a big part of your life. I was just wondering what you're next project was going to be?"

I hesitated.

"I don't know," I said.

CHAPTER SIXTY-EIGHT

After the funeral I immersed myself in my remaining rotations -
I told myself my relation with the family was over, and I
shouldn't try to hold on.

A few weeks later, though, I had the urge to phone Shoniah.

"Oh, I'm okay," she said, and laughed endearingly. "Did you
hear the news?"

"No," I said. "What?"

"Auntie Belle died...

"She had a cold the week before. When I called her the other day
and she didn't answer, I knew...

"They told us her death was probably because of her heart..."

The funeral was held in the Sunnyside church Auntie Belle had
attended for fifty years.

Samuel went to the pulpit.

"She was a woman of few words." Then his features softened,
and emanated a gentle glow. "And, you know, it's the quiet people
who often say the most - *Just with their silence...*"

The preacher rose, and planted his hands firmly on the pulpit -

"She had no children!" he bellowed in a stirring voice. "But she
was..."

I shook my head.

No, I thought. She did have a child.

Auntie Belle was buried close to Ethel...

Shoniah and Karl invited me to their home.

They lived in a suburb twenty miles northeast of Streeport.

As I pulled into the driveway their dog chased the rope dangling from the front of my car.

"Mike, what's that?!" Karl laughed.

"Part of the fender tore off," I said.

"When did that happen?"

"The night of the flood."

"Oh."

He was quiet.

I went into the house.

Karl stayed behind, and examined the damage...

"I should have known," I told Shoniah. "I should have known how Ethel's passing would affect her..."

"I don't think there's anything you could have done," she said. "It's not like people weren't around her. I saw her a lot. She was still taking care of Sammy..."

I went out.

Karl was resetting the fender.

"I attached some binders to it, Mike. I think that should hold it...

"Hey, Mike, I have to pick up some food for dinner. You want to come?..."

The shopping mall was a short drive from the house.

"I like it out here," Karl said. "Everything you need is close."

We picked out some hamburger, and brought it to the checkout counter.

"Karl, I'd like to pay for this - I appreciate you fixing my car, and want to repay you..."

"No, Mike," he laughed. "You've done enough..."

I met Dr. Hood passing through the corridors of Claude Ray.

"You look much better!" he said.

I nodded.

"Oh, yeah. It just looks like a weight's been taken off of your shoulders!..."

"Thank you," I said.

As I walked past a concerned look gripped his features.

"Are you okay?"

"Where is the line," I thought, "between true concern and a clinician's ploy to ferret something out of you?"

"Yes, I'm okay, Dr. Hood. Thank you..."

I went to Miami, where I used to stay with my grandparents, and worked at the Jackson Memorial Hospital -

Then, to New York, where I stayed with family, and worked at Harlem Hospital.

But even as graduation neared, I didn't have any plans.

"Something I might enjoy," I told my friend Eric, "is taking a course in massage. There were so many times I'd be massaging Ethel, thinking, 'If only I had some formal training, I'd be able to help her so much better.'"

"Why don't you come back to California, and take a massage course out here?" he said. "I know a massage school that offers a month long intensive - Great way to learn about yourself..."

I called the school, and made arrangements to attend...

In the hallway of The Marymount I passed John Wang.

"Hey, how you doing?" he said. "How is that friend of yours we met that day outside Claude Ray?"

"She died," I said. "I miss her."

John assumed a thoughtful pose.

"Plato said that the highest form of friendship is that relationship where neither party wants or has something to gain from the other...

"Lower forms, you're in it for what the other person can give you."

I smiled and shook my head.

"They're not bad," he said. "We all have relationships like that - You need them - They're necessary.

"I mean, let's face it. Your friend is gone, and you're in the same place you were before you met her... She didn't give you anything..."

That weekend Ethel's family invited me to their home.

They lived in what Ethel referred to as "the country", about an hours' ride west of Streeport.

On the way over I got lost, and parked to the side of the road and looked at a map.

A car pulled up next of me - The people inside laughing.

"You lost, Mike?!" Ethel's niece Gina called out, grinning to the others.

"Yes, I am."

"Well, follow us, then!..."

Mr. Small led me inside his home.

"Mike, I want you to treat this place like your own house."

He opened the door to a secluded room.

"There will always be a room for you here."

"And those aren't just words from the mouth," he said. "They come from the heart..."

Mrs. Small lay on the couch, just released from the hospital after another bout of pneumonia.

"Hi Mikie. How you doing, sugar?... Go get yourself something to eat."

Dishes and platters filled the table.

I eyed the barbecued ribs -

"They're so good, Mike," Ethel had told me. "They literally melt in your mouth..."

"Oh, come on, Ethel," I'd said. "Ribs don't melt in your mouth."

"They do, Mike. They melt in your mouth."

I turned to Mr. Small.

"I hear ribs are your specialty."

"Yeah. I's make them by soaking them in barbecue sauce for a few days - Then I's prepare them in my pit - It has a furnace on the one side, and a place for the meat on the other. There's a hole in between that lets the smoke go through and heat the meat. I let them cook that way for a couple more days - Sometimes three."

I bit into the rib -

It dissolved before I could chew it.

It did! I thought. It did! It melts in your mouth!

I had never believed her - No matter how many times she'd told me.

"That's amazing," I said...

A large affable man greeted me on the porch.

"Hi," he said, shaking my hand. "I'm Lionel - Isaiah's son."

Lionel was a baker, and a preacher.

"I like helping the homeless," he said. "There's this one guy I hand out change to - He sits in the middle of the street - I know that every time he sees my white Buick drive up his eyes light up because he knows his meal ticket's comin'...

"Well, one day I'm driving by this guy, and I was about to give him some change, when God says to me, 'Five dollars'.

"'Five dollars?!', I say. 'Gees, isn't that a bit much?!'

"Well, right afterwards, I get to the bakery and find out we'd just been contracted for a $1500 deal - That five dollars was no problem."

"I heard a story recently," I said. "A patient told me one night he was driving home on a secluded stretch of farm road. He kept a CB radio in his car, and, from out of the blue, God called him on it.

"'After this accident you're about to get into,' God says, 'use the CB to call for assistance because there won't be time to wait for the ambulance.'

"'No I ain't!', he says, and slams on the brakes.

"Just as his car comes to a grinding halt, another comes barreling in out of nowhere - Crosses right in front of him - Missing his car by inches - Then crashes into an embankment.

"Now, what I find so provocative about his story is this - If God is omniscient, how is it that my patient was literally able to steer clear of something God had predicted?"

"Well, you do have a Will." His tone was matter-of-fact, as though the answer were obvious. "What I was telling you before about the five dollars - That was just a voice in my head. I could choose to listen, or I could have chose not to...

"You do have a Will..."

Ethel's older brother, Clyde, arrived at the house.

He'd worn an eye patch at the funeral; now, the patch was gone, revealing a scarred left eye.

He went stumbling through the kitchen, terrorizing Lionel's five year old son, little Isaiah.

"What'chu afraid of?!" he shouted. *"I'm gonna take it out! What'chu running away from?!"*

"Stop it, Clyde!" the boy cried. *"Stop!"*

The little boy ran between the adults.

His younger sister slapped at Clyde's leg.

"No, Clyde! No!"

Clyde kept taunting little Isaiah until he had him cornered between a closet and the refrigerator -

"Why you crying like that?! You scared of this?! What you crying for?! Ahh!"

Clyde moved off.

The little boy stood reduced to tears.

"What's the matter?" I said.

"He's scaring me," he cried.

Tears welled up in my eyes.

"He hurt his eye," I said. "It's like a scar - But instead of skin, it's over his eye -

"It must have hurt a lot..."

Clyde came back in the kitchen.

"You still scared... I'll take it out..."

Isaiah stood looking at him - And didn't call out, or run away...

It was dark, and Mr. Small walked me to my car.

"I really enjoyed the party, Mr. Small. Especially, your ribs - Ethel had told me so much about them."

"Yeah. She really enjoyed that. You had the food we cooked over Christmas?"

"No. I was away on the east coast."

"Oh." He looked away. "I barbecued a turkey then."

"Ethel told me. She said she wished I was there - Just so I could taste all the foods and enjoy the smells - 'They were so flavorful,' she said."

"Yeah. She enjoyed that - I miss her."

"I do, too..."

"But we all gotta go sometime."

"Yes. Something to look forward to - Seeing her again."

"Yeah. That's true."

He stood planted, and his face lost all expression.

"Are you alright, Mr. Small?"

"Oh, yeah," he said with a start. "I was just thinking about you... I was thinking how good you were to her..."

Clyde ambled towards us.

"Whoo-wee! We can't get rid of this boy?" He curled his arm around my neck, and leaned into me. "Who you in love with? Who're you in love with?"

He slipped a beer into my hand.

"Hey, you want this?... No, you don't want that?!" He looked over at Mr. Small. "You see that?!"

Mr. Small looked down and shook his head.

"You alright," Clyde said. "Love ya, brother."

He hugged me. He was big and muscular the way Matthew was, but his hands were swollen, like a pair of inflated gloves.

"You take care now," he said, and went stumbling into the night.

"The most important thing," Mr. Small said, "is to be loved."

He looked in Clyde's direction.

"If you're not loved by someone," he said, choking on the words. "You're pitiful..."

CHAPTER SIXTY-NINE

I met Chris in front of the security booth after the funeral.

"Hey, I was thinking of that friend of yours - the young woman with cancer. How is she?"

"She passed," I said.

"Oh, I'm sorry to hear that." He put his head down. *"Were you with her?"*

"Yes," I said. "It was pretty tough. A lot of things went wrong that night. I was trying to help her, but I'm afraid I might have made her suffering worse..."

"Let me tell you something," he said. *"There wasn't anything you did wrong. It was her time to go, and nothing you could have done would have mattered or made any difference. Sometimes you have to accept that God has a plan for all of us, and when it's your time there's nothing any of us can do.*

"You just have to accept God's will."

I nodded.

"Chris, can I tell you something?"

"Yeah, sure, man. What's that?"

"On the night of her death her heart kept beating, even after her last breath. I stood there waiting for it to stop - It never did."

Chris drew himself up, and put his hand to his chin.

"How do I say this respectfully - The way I see it, she hadn't left you yet - She was still in that room with you - She didn't want to leave you."

I looked away.

"Did you at any time feel her hand twitch, or move, or something like that?"

His voice was timid, and the question caught me by surprise -

"No," I said, startled. "There wasn't anything like that..."

Then I looked at him -

"But, you know, Chris, when I finally went to let go, it was like she was still holding on to me - I literally had to pull my hand out of her grasp."

Chris shook his head and smiled - Then laughed and stamped his feet -

"I don't know," he said. "I think you really loved that woman - And she really loved you. Who knows? Maybe, you would have got married."

"All I know," he said, with broad smile and radiant expression. "Is I look forward to a time - when I see you - And your heart is full of joy. I think she'd like that, too like that, too...."

THE END

ABOUT THE AUTHOR

Michael Yanuck MD PhD is a physician-scientist
whose groundbreaking research at the National Institutes of
Health was the basis for a FDA-approved vaccine for cancer.
Following a traumatic leg injury he returned to medicine. Intent on
caring for the less fortunate, he enlisted in the National Health
Service Corps, worked in urban and rural health centers throughout
the country, then served native peoples with the Indian Health
Service. Now, he cares for homeless Veterans at the Sacramento VA
Medical Center, as well as serves as Pain Champion for all of
Northern California. He continues to perform bioenergy,
which he teaches to the public.

www.ingramcontent.com/pod-product-compliance
Lightning Source LLC
Chambersburg PA
CBHW031317040426
42443CB00005B/106